BREATHE AGAIN NATURALLY

How to Deal with Catarrh, Bronchitis, Asthma & Manage Lung and Bronchial Problems Through A Natural Living & Eating Program

by BERNARD JENSEN, DC
Nutritionist

The information in this book is presented for educational purposes only. It consists of the best information available to the author, and is based on many years of study, experience and research throughout the world. This information is not intended to be used for diagnostic purposes for any individual or condition except by a qualified health professional. In every case where a specific health problem exists, competent professional advice should be sought.

FIRST EDITION

Published by
Bernard Jensen Enterprises
24360 Old Wagon Road
Escondido, California 92027

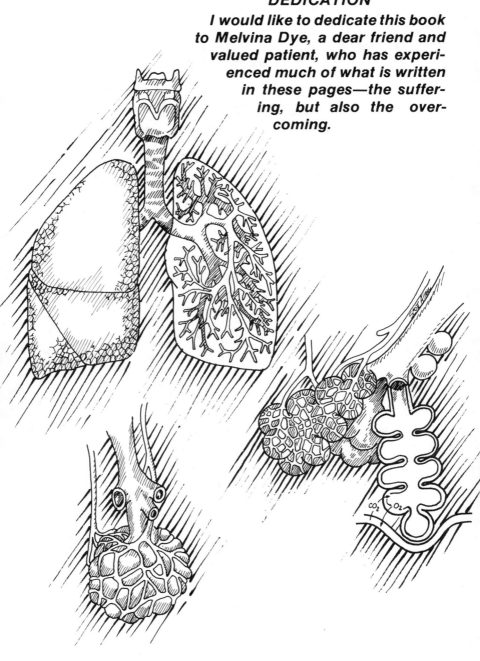

CONTENTS

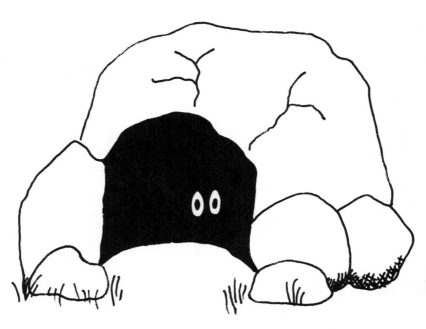

"The Bear Awakens!"

Prefatory Author's Note

We have considered asthma as the primary subject of this book because it is the most difficult respiratory case to handle. Yet before asthma develops, it is preceded by many lesser respiratory problems—colds, flu, tonsillitis, coughs, allergies, pneumonia and bronchial troubles. If we can get rid of the asthma, all the others will disappear.

On the other hand, by using the same reversal process applied to asthma in this book on any of the lesser stages of respiratory problems, we can get rid of them, and asthma will not develop.

In over fifty years of sanitarium practice, I have found a parallel condition always associated with respiratory disease. Bowel troubles always precede and accompany respiratory conditions. The bowel is one of the most important parts of the body, and unless it is taken care of, the respiratory condition, whether acute or chronic, will remain and grow worse.

Iris analysis shows that inherent weakness of the lungs or bronchials is inevitably linked with inherent weakness of the colon. Perhaps 98% of my patients have had potential or actual bronchial problems, as revealed in the iris.

I know what respiratory problems are like because I have experienced them myself. My mother died of tuberculosis when I was young, and I inherited her respiratory weakness. In my teens, trying to gain weight by drinking as many malts as possible, I developed a bronchial condition which the doctors said was rapidly turning into bronchiectosis. They had no cure for it. The doctors gave up and told me to go home and go to bed. I was stunned. How could they tell a person to give up?

Determined to fight the problem, I learned breathing exercises from Dr. Thomas Gaines, putting four inches on my chest in a year's time. I began looking into nutrition and other nature cure arts. From what I learned, I have been able to leave my respiratory condition behind and help thousands of others over the years, realizing that health is a way of life, not simply an occasional remedial effort when dis-ease rears its ugly head.

I want you—the reader—to know that respiratory conditions can be overcome—nature's way—if you have the determination, diligence and patience to do it.

INTRODUCTION

Advanced respiratory conditions—asthma, bronchitis and other such diseases—are among the most difficult of all health problems to take care of, generally because they have taken many years to develop, and catarrhal settlements are deeply embedded in the tissues. Yet, I have seen many patients emerge victorious from the battle, leaving their drugs, atomizers and inhalers behind after following nature's way of cleansing and rejuvenating the body. Although we focus primarily on asthma in this book, the same principles can be applied to any chronic respiratory problem.

Asthma is like grabbing a bear by the tail—the cure (letting go) is almost worse than the condition (holding on).

I dread seeing an asthma patient walk in my office door because I know what we're both going to have to go through if he or she is really serious about getting rid of it. When an asthma victim follows the natural healing program I teach, he goes through a series of healing crises. These resemble his past asthma attacks so much that the patient often panics, even when he has been forewarned what to expect.

The good news is that asthma can be overcome. No more racking cough, no more wheezing and gasping, no more terrifying experiences of near suffocation. Not temporary relief, permanent relief!

Like Rome, no chronic respiratory disease was built in a day, and many factors may contribute to its development. Genetic inheritance (inherent weaknesses), environment, home life, diet, personal habits, attitudes and emotional responses (psychosomatic causes)—all these and more can contribute.

Catarrh is the first and universal sign of disease preconditions in the body, a sign that something is wrong, that tissue irritation is present. Catarrh is the excess mucus secreted by irritated tissue, and it shows up before anything else, before we can name a disease or condition. **ALL RESPIRATORY CONDITIONS ARE**

CATARRHAL CONDITIONS. WHETHER THE PROBLEM MANIFESTS AS A COLD, FLU, ASTHMA OR OTHER CONDITION, IT IS STILL A CATARRHAL PROBLEM.

Disease goes through four typical stages, all representing the body's attempt to get rid of catarrh that has been driven deeply into the tissues. The acute stage of respiratory disease begins with coughs, fevers, colds, flu, allergies and all the "itises," such as tonsillitis, laryngitis, sinusitis and bronchitis. The subacute and chronic stages may still include any of the "itises," which become progressively more serious with time. Typical subacute problems are hay fever and sinus trouble, while at the chronic stage we often find pneumonia, asthma and bronchitis. Emphysema is the final, degenerative stage.

What we need to understand is that we don't "catch" diseases, we create them by the way we live.

Bronchitis, hay fever and asthma symptoms are not infrequently found in children. We find that children may outgrow these at puberty when hormonal changes alter the body chemistry and stimulate growth. If they do not, then the condition will become more advanced and chronic until after some years a semi-invalid or invalid stage is reached. That is, unless they change the life patterns contributing to the condition.

Asthma is characterized by spasms of the bronchial tubes associated with congestion caused by catarrh, mucus and phlegm accumulated over a long period of time. Chronic bronchitis is an inflammation of the bronchi, an outgrowth of years of tissue irritation and catarrhal suppression. Its onset is usually in middle-age or later, and symptoms include difficulty in breathing, shortness of breath, constant coughing, expectoration of phlegm and frequent infections in the bronchial tubes. Suppression or control of symptoms like runny nose, itchy eyes, sneezing and fever by drugs, atomizers and inhalants drives catarrh "underground," so to speak, causing it to build up in tissues. To get rid of asthma or bronchitis, we have to get rid of old catarrhal accumulations by strengthening the health of the entire body and by eliminating as many of the contributing causes as possible.

This brings us to the reversal process. Hering's law of cure states, ***"All cure starts from within out and from the head down, in reverse order as the symptoms first appeared."*** As the patient gains strength, new tissue grows in place of the old, and a healing crisis develops. Old catarrh, phlegm and toxic accumulations are purged from the body.

What happens if chronic respiratory disease isn't taken care of? As I stated before, it can degenerate into emphysema. Emphysema is the end of the road, the point at which the alveoli or air sacs of the lungs have become seriously compromised. I have helped a few emphysema patients regain their health, but for others, it was too late. They had already bought their tickets to the "other side."

For those who have truly "let go of the bear's tail," life is a joy again, almost beyond belief. With old, unhealthy habits discarded, a new path lies ahead—a higher path. Health is not, as some say, freedom from disease. It is a joyful way of life.

It is difficult to realize what a pall is cast over life by the constant battle against chronic respiratory disease until a person has won that battle and is free. The sky is blue again, the sunshine is warm and wonderful, the gentle breeze caresses the skin and the perfume of beautiful flowers floats on the air! Life is good!

A word of warning to the patient. This book is in no way intended to take the place of your doctor. Asthma and other chronic lung conditions are serious business, and any effort to treat them should be done under medical supervision.

> *"It seems to me that those sciences which are not born of experience, the mother of all certainty, and which do not end in known experience—that is to say, those sciences whose origin or process or end does not pass through any of the five senses—are vain and full of errors."*
>
> —Leonardo Da Vinci

PART I. CATCHING A BEAR BY THE TAIL

Chapter 1. Catarrh—On the Trail

Catarrh is the universal sign of disease or disease-producing processes at work in the body. It always signals that we are on the trail of some condition we would prefer to avoid, and it is inevitably present in all respiratory conditions.

Catarrh comes from the Greek words *cata* (down) and *rhein* (flow)—to flow down. It refers to the mucus produced under conditions of tissue inflammation. The presence of catarrh signals the onset of a cold, flu or other condition, and our usual response is to run to the drugstore and buy something to suppress it. Has anyone ever considered that catarrhal elimination might be a **natural lifesaving process**?

Catarrh is not so much a cause of disease conditions as it is a sign that tissue inflammation exists in the body. That is, it is a result of tissue inflammation which, in turn, is a result of some form of irritation. We find that many different substances and processes can irritate tissue.

Under normal conditions mucus is produced by goblet cells in the mucus membranes lining the alimentary system, the respiratory system and parts of the genito-urinary system. Its functions are lubrication and protection. Foreign particles, bacteria and other substances are usually prevented from reaching the sensitive mucous membrane by entrapment in the sticky mucus, which carries them away.

For example, normally mucus developed in the bronchial tubes is moved along continuously by ciliary action until it is expelled through the mouth and nose. When the tissue becomes irritated and inflamed, perhaps due to exposure to an allergen, the mucus flow increases to assist in carrying off the source of irritation. This increased mucus flow is called catarrh. The gathering catarrh reduces the size of air passages which causes a strain on the alveoli of the lungs where the oxygen/carbon dioxide exchange takes place.

A cough is Nature's way of clearing catarrh from the throat and bronchial areas. A deep inspiration is followed by the closure of the glottis and vocal cords over the trachea. As the diaphragm relaxes, the stomach and chest muscles contract, building up pressure in the chest. The resulting blast of air helps dislodge any catarrh, phlegm or mucus. Coughing increases according to the degree of chronicity, since the tissue softens and ciliary action diminishes with time.

WHAT IS A "CATARRHAL CONDITION?"

What we term a catarrhal condition is Nature's method of ridding the body of ingested irritants or internally-produced wastes not taken care of in the normal elimination process. When catarrhal elimination reaches the "running" stage, that means the body is waging a real battle to get rid of some unwanted substance before it can harm the tissues.

The elimination should never be stopped by suppressant drugs or other treatment, or the catarrh carrying the irritating substance will be forced to remain in the body. Any discharge from the body is a natural effort to get rid of something that does not belong there. It is a cleansing process aimed at getting rid of toxic settlements before they thicken, harden and settle into the inherently weak organs or tissues of the body.

A disease condition may be divided into four stages from the time of onset: acute, subacute, chronic and degenerative. The acute stage is the "running" stage, the time when the body is actively trying to throw off toxins or wastes. If we use unnatural methods to stop these acute processes of elimination, they will develop into subacute stages.

The body's normal defenses act as a police department to keep order. When we stop a catarrhal discharge we have not effected a cure or conquered a disease. We have merely prolonged the day of reckoning.

WHY DO CATARRHAL CONDITIONS DEVELOP?

There are probably hundreds of little reasons why catarrhal conditions develop, but the basic causes are two. The body is constantly changing, growing, exchanging new cells for old in obedience to the basic law of life. This means the thousands of life processes in the body are all moving, all flowing. Movement is life; stagnation is death. When any life process slows down to a certain point, tissue irritation takes place, inflammation arises and catarrh develops.

In other words, a living organism such as man is a dynamic complex of powerful electro-chemical processes, a factory where vital functions are being carried out every second. You cannot stop any of these processes or functions without causing damage somewhere in the organism. If nutrients are stopped, cells starve, die and almost immediately begin to decompose. This decomposition irritates neighboring tissue, causes inflammation and there we go again. If the movement of metabolic wastes is halted, this strongly acidic material immediately begins to irritate the surrounding tissue. Of course, bacteria and viruses feed on and multiply in dead tissue of any kind. Germ life thrives on stagnation while dramatically increasing inflammation. The law of life is flow, movement, dynamism, and we must remember it.

Genetic factors make up the second important cause. Everyone is born with certain strengths and weaknesses in the anatomy and physiology of the body. The strengths take care of themselves, so it is the weaknesses with which we must be concerned, because these are the areas of the body that will cause us trouble. A chain is only as strong as its weakest link, and the same principle applies to the human body.

An inherent weakness in the body may be defined as an organ or tissue area with an underactive metabolism. That is, nutrients are not assimilated and wastes are not eliminated as efficiently as in other organs and tissues. A sudden chill, overwork or inadequate diet would affect this part of the body more severely than other parts.

If we know we have an inherently weak colon or bronchial area, we should as a matter of common sense guard against conditions that would harm them. We should avoid overexerting ourselves to the point of straining the lungs and we should avoid constipating foods, for example. Simply put, we need to be aware of our inherent weaknesses and take care of them.

We find that the sensitivity of inherently weak tissue to irritation is greater than that of normal tissue. Inflammation is more easily produced and remains longer, which means that catarrh is a more serious problem in areas of inherent weakness. Unless the strength of these weaker body areas is maintained by an informed and vital approach to health, they may easily become repositories for catarrhal settlements, drug or chemical residues and other toxic wastes. It doesn't take much to reduce the metabolic efficiency of an inherently weak organ to the point where it is unable, of its own power, to throw off toxic wastes.

Asthma represents such a weakened state in the respiratory system. Asthma attacks are the feeble efforts of a weakened lung structure to rid itself of catarrhal encumbrances. It can't be done—not without strengthening the respiratory system first.

One of the most common reasons for the existence of catarrh in any part of the body is fatigue. A tired body develops acids which irritate the mucous membranes. The fatigue may be due to work habits which place undue strain on certain portions of the body. Catarrh can be produced by overeating; using wrong food combinations over long periods of time; the use of narcotics, drugs, tobacco, etc.; anything that violates the equilibrium of the body or saps its strength.

It isn't what we do once in a while that counts—it's what we do most of the time—our patterns of living. A person who breaks the law for the first time may be let off with a light fine or punishment as a one-time offender. But, if we continue to break the law, we will end up with a long prison term, large fine or both.

Catching a cold is no serious matter, but if we continue habitually in the behavior pattern that brought it on, we will eventually develop a chronic condition. If we have already become habitual offenders against the law of Nature, then it is up to us to correct our habits and try to establish law and order again.

STARTING OFF RIGHT

Most ill health in adults has its roots in childhood. Colds and children's diseases such as mumps, measles, ear infections and tonsillitis should be taken care of by natural methods. We should remember that cleanliness, correct foods, stimulating activities and a happy environment with plenty of love will prevent most ill health in children. Even those with inherent weaknesses will—if properly cared for—escape most childhood diseases and become healthy adults.

Children do not naturally take care of themselves or develop good health habits. If they are having fun, they will nonchalantly skip a bowel movement or forget to eat lunch. Children do not know their limits for overexertion, fatigue or staying up too late. They violate Nature's laws with innocent impunity.

It is the parents' job to see that their children develop good health habits—whether they appreciate what you do or not.

SYMPTOMS

It is possible to innocently break a law which we do not realize exists until we are caught by a policeman. "Ignorance of the law is no excuse," says the judge. It may seem harsh, but the idea is the protection of the public.

The body also has its policemen who warn us when we are breaking the law. They are known as "symptoms." Symptoms are in the form of discharges, pains, aches and inflammations which occur when something is wrong in the body.

We find that symptoms usually appear first in the mucus membranes. They grow more serious as we continue violating Nature's laws until the body has a major breakdown.

The progression from colds and flu to hay fever and sinus trouble to bronchitis and asthma is a perfect example. The progression is generally due to suppressive methods of treatment.

A weakened body and sluggish blood and lymph circulation react to every change in temperature. Every little breeze that blows becomes an ill wind. What should be normal adjustments to changing weather (temperature, humidity, atmospheric pressure) become violent reactions. We can't take them in stride.

We get summer colds, winter colds, attacks of asthma, hay fever, sinusitis and bronchitis.

These are the symptoms of acute and subacute conditions, the result of neglecting earlier symptoms or of suppressing catarrhal elimination.

It is vitally important for me to impress upon you the harm you do your body and the misery you are setting yourself up for when

you suppress colds and other mino
lesson, then you are on your way

Nervousness and depression
catarrhal conditions. Stress, ter
likelihood of disease and redu
recuperate, so we have to deal
stress and disease are a chicken-
produce more of the other.

Catarrhal suppression and
in the direction of chronic disea
in the direction of better health. In U..,
titled "Pathways to Health and Disease" in whicn we
development of chronic disease and how to reverse it. But it we
learn to bear with the aches, pains and discomforts of the body's
natural cleansing processes, we can avoid chronic conditions and
move in the direction of vital well-being.

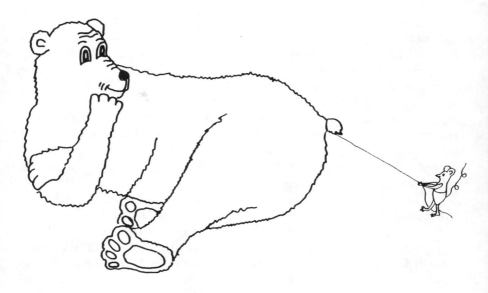

Asthma, hay fever and chronic bronchitis are like catching a bear by the tail. The question is, what are you going to do with that bear?

Chapter 2. Bronchitis and Asthma Country

To catch a bear, so they say, you have to know something about the country bears live in. The same is true of asthma and bronchitis, which are disorders of the respiratory system.

YOUR RESPIRATORY SYSTEM

Respiration, the process of taking air into the lungs and then expelling it, brings life-giving oxygen to the body and expels carbon dioxide and other gases. Oxygen is vital to all metabolism, especially in the brain.

Our respiratory system is made up of the nose, throat, larynx, windpipe and lungs. The lungs, which nearly fill the chest, are constructed like two inverted trees: the right and left bronchi, air passages from the trachea, form the trunks; bronchioles form the branches; and at the ends of all bronchioles are the "leaves," the alveoli or air sacs. It is in the alveoli where oxygen is exchanged for carbon dioxide.

The entire respiratory system is lined with mucus membrane, lubricated by mucus secreted from small glands under the surface. The mucus not only lubricates the membrane but protects it, capturing the dust particles and microorganisms we breathe in. Larger foreign particles are filtered out of the air we breathe by the hairs in the nose. The rest are caught in the sticky mucus lining and expelled by special cells called cilia which move the mucus out. Sneezing and coughing are reflex activities designed to expel mucus.

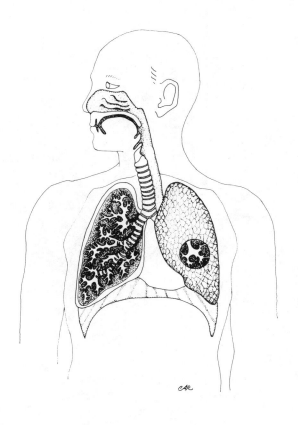

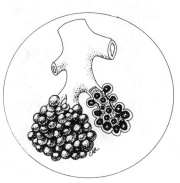

The respiratory system, with enlarged view of the alveoli or air sacs of the lungs, where oxygen is exchanged for carbon dioxide. The lungs are the only organs which assimilate a vital nutrient and expel waste through the same passage ways.

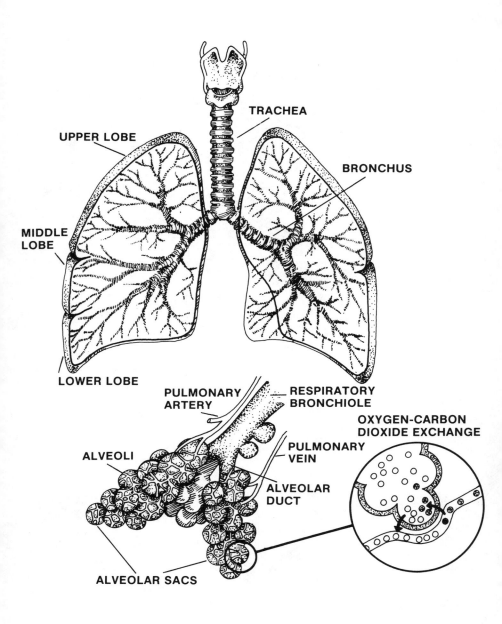

TRACHEA

UPPER LOBE

BRONCHUS

MIDDLE
LOBE

LOWER LOBE

PULMONARY
ARTERY

RESPIRATORY
BRONCHIOLE

OXYGEN-CARBON
DIOXIDE EXCHANGE

ALVEOLI

PULMONARY
VEIN

ALVEOLAR
DUCT

ALVEOLAR SACS

Upper view: Bronchial "tree" of the lungs, showing structural arrangement of respiratory passages. Lower left: The alveoli or air sacs are at the ends of the small bronchi, like small clusters of grapes. Lower right: Schematic view of oxygen-carbon dioxide exchange between air sacs and a blood capillary.

12

The sinuses, hollows in the facial bones, also help keep the nasal passages moist. The sinuses have only one opening, and when the mucus membrane swells enough to close it, the internal pressure can be very painful.

The normal breathing rate for a resting adult is about 16-20 times/minute; for a child, it is around 25-30 times/minute. The air we inhale is 21% oxygen, 79% nitrogen, 0.04% carbon dioxide. Exhaled air is 16% oxygen, 79.5% nitrogen and 4% carbon dioxide. Our lungs use about one-fourth of the oxygen we inhale.

Surrounding and protecting the lungs is the bony "cage" called the thorax, made up of ribs, cartilage, breastbone and backbone. The intercostal muscles expand and contract the rib cage when we breathe. Correct posture when we stand or sit is important to full, free breathing.

A "normal" breath by a person not involved in physical activity might be a pint or less of air. The deepest breath we can take, after forcing out all possible air, is about one gallon in volume. Relaxed breathing is full and deep. A fearful or anxious person breathes rapidly and shallowly.

The respiratory center of the brain is the medulla, which also controls heart rate and many of the digestive functions via the vagus nerve. Our limited voluntary control of breathing comes from the cerebral cortex. Special nerve ends in the carotid and aortic bodies sense changes in blood pressure or acidity and adjust respiration to compensate. The important thing to notice is that breathing, heart rate, digestion, blood chemistry and brain function are all connected.

Of course, the correct functioning of the respiratory system requires that we have good health habits—proper diet, posture, exercise, fresh air, sunshine, relaxation, rest and attitudes. Emotions such as fear or anger affect the breathing much differently than love or joy, as we all know. We exercise a great deal of control over these things, and it is usually our fault if they are neglected.

Other things, we find, are beyond our control. You may have inherited a weak lung structure or a sluggish bowel that continually allows toxins to filter into the bloodstream. You may have inherited allergy problems from one or both parents. You may live in a city where the air is polluted by auto exhaust emissions and industrial chemicals. The fruit and vegetables you buy may have been grown in depleted soils. Your nerves may be jangled by the noise, pace and pressures of modern living.

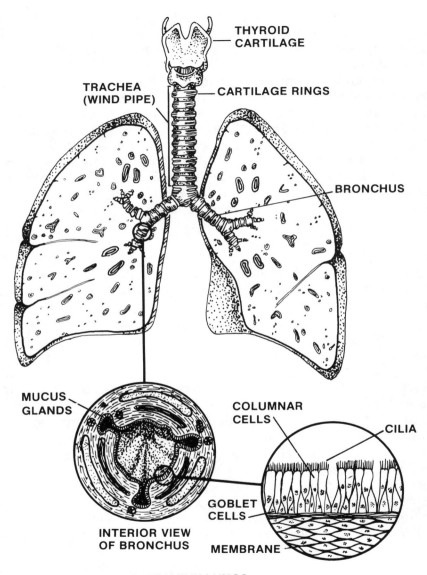

THYROID CARTILAGE

TRACHEA (WIND PIPE)

CARTILAGE RINGS

BRONCHUS

MUCUS GLANDS

COLUMNAR CELLS

CILIA

GOBLET CELLS

INTERIOR VIEW OF BRONCHUS

MEMBRANE

HEALTHY LUNGS

The bronchi or air passages of the lungs are self-cleaning by means of the cilia (enlarged insets), soft "micro-brushes" that sweep catarrh, mucus, dust and other foreign matter up toward the throat where a cough can expel it. Smoking coats the cilia with tar and can delay expulsion of catarrh and toxic waste substances for up to two years.

You may have adopted poor health habits out of ignorance. The cure for ignorance is education and study. (If you are a junk food junkie or a sugar addict, kick the habit now that you know better. Find out the right way to live and follow that path.)

Now that we have explored the country inhabited by asthma, let's look at a sample case.

STEP 1 FROM COLDS AND FLUS TO CHRONIC RESPIRATORY PROBLEMS

The first step toward any chronic disease, as discussed in Chapter 1, is the development of tissue inflammation and the subsequent production of catarrh. The sensitivity of the respiratory tract and its role in catarrhal elimination make it vulnerable to many sources of irritation, internal as well as external, particularly if the sinuses, bronchi or lungs are inherently weak structures to begin with.

Internal sources of irritation include the waste acids produced in the process of metabolism. Stress can result in the production of excess nerve acids, while fatigue is a state in which acids due to muscular activity or gastrointestinal function are not neutralized and carried away as fast as they are formed. Even normal metabolic wastes may accumulate to excess if the eliminative channels are not working efficiently. An underactive bowel is nearly always found in combination with lung or bronchial weaknesses. Because the tonsils are lymphatic tissue, any overloading of the lymphatic system with acids or other toxic substances can bring on irritation and inflammation of the tonsils—tonsillitis. If the source of tonsillitis is not taken care of, the toxic irritation of the tonsils may spread to the sinuses, nasal passages and bronchi.

We find that external irritants to the respiratory system range from dust and pollen particles to foods. How can foods irritate the respiratory system? There are two ways. First, foods that irritate the stomach—such as chocolate, the juice of unripe oranges, coffee and others—may reflexly irritate the lungs via the vagus nerve, which serves the mucous membrane of the larynx, trachea, bronchi and lungs as well as the esophagus and stomach. Some functions involving this nerve are coughing, sneezing, swallowing, secretions from the glands of the stomach and pancreas, and the sensation of hunger. The functions of the respiratory system are intimately connected with the digestive system through the vagus nerve.

Secondly, undigested food substances are treated as waste products and may load up the lymphatic system, leading to irritation of the tonsils and mucous membranes of the throat. Digestion is poor when we are tired, and we should never eat a heavy meal at that time. Persons lacking hydrochloric acid in the stomach cannot completely digest proteins. Milk, chocolate and wheat products are heavy catarrh producers in many people. Some foods may also cause an allergic reaction.

What we breathe affects our respiratory system. Obviously toxic examples are smog and coal dust. Coal miners, after working many years in the mines, may come up with pneumoconiosis, a lung disease directly caused by prolonged irritation of the lung tissue by coal dust. Smokers are prone to a high incidence of lung and throat cancer because the toxins in tobacco smoke cannot be eliminated as fast as they are introduced into the body. The same principle applies to anything we inhale—dust, pollens, smog, fumes from paint, dyes, photographic chemicals, solvents, glue, epoxy resins and many other substances. These irritate the respiratory system lining and may interact chemically with it or with other substances in the lymph or blood.

Researchers have found that those who get tuberculosis are frequently in a low state of resistance—fatigued, under stress, malnourished or weakened from other illnesses. At that point, a person exposed to tuberculosis bacilli can get the disease. The important point to notice here is that the disease cannot take hold until the lungs are in a weakened condition, through incorrect eating and living patterns. In my view, the weakening of the lung structure may lead to any of several chronic respiratory problems, and we cannot be sure what it will be.

When a person uses foods that do not nourish the body, chemical shortages begin to show up. Asthma, bronchitis and other respiratory conditions may start with a lack of potassium. Potassium is one of the great alkalizers in the body, and we must have plenty of it throughout our lives.

Potassium is found in greens and in raw vegetables. Few people eat enough of these foods, especially early in life.

The patients I treat tell me about the difficulty they have with their children's eating habits: they won't eat salads or certain vegetables and fruits, but they do like certain things such as sweets, as a rule. The mother, the housewife, gives in to the child's likes and dislikes rather than having them eat what is good for them. Sweets are used for bribery. "If you eat your spinach, you can have a cookie."

Foods that lack substance for the body but are full of calories begin to interact with the inherent weaknesses, those organs and tissues which are structurally deficient.

These early years of shortages are compounded when a child reaches school age, because the lunches served by the schools are often seriously inadequate. Limited finances force the schools to serve cheap commercially-processed foods. By adding chemical preservatives, companies can put "eternal life" into a food, allowing it to sit in warehouses or on store shelves for long periods of time until it is bought by the consumer. Longer shelf life lowers the price. Because we are bargain minded, we get the cheapest foods we can live on. But, we pay for it in other ways.

Before we realize it, we are members of the Junk Food Club. The body's innate intelligence rebels against membership, and we enter the "Age of Colds," runny nose, nasal congestion and sneezing.

STEP 2: THE AGE OF COLDS

During the age of colds, mother heads for the drugstore and brings home cold remedies, cough syrups, Formula X-123...almost all of which are suppressants. She doesn't want her child to suffer needlessly, and something has to be found to stop that cold overnight.

The child is back in school the next day with the cold under control. But, a price has been paid to get rid of the symptoms. The congestion and toxic wastes that the body was trying to eliminate are still there.

After it is prevented from flowing, catarrh settles into the body, migrating to the inherent weaknesses. Stronger organs and tissues have the capacity to resist and throw off toxic wastes. Weak ones do not.

The catarrhal settlement naturally irritates the mucus membrane and a little bronchial cough develops. Mother brings out a super-suppressant cough syrup, the cough is stopped and the catarrh settles deeper. If it flares up again, it is suppressed again. As time goes on, the catarrh moves deeper and deeper into the lung structure.

STEP 3: FLU

Flu, which is short for influenza, follows the "age of colds," bringing longer periods of discomfort and requiring stronger drugs to suppress. We stop the flu the same way we stopped the colds—with chemical suppressants.

Mother still serves the same foods at mealtimes and the children snack on chocolate, cookies, milk and other catarrh-forming foods in between meals. We may be encouraged to overeat or to eat poor food combinations. There may be little variety in the diet, few fresh fruits and vegetables.

The flu strikes again, and this time the drugstore remedies aren't effective. So, we head for the doctor's office. Returning home with a powerful prescription drug, we still have to spend some time in bed.

Each time the flu returns, we have a tougher time with it. We have not heeded Nature's warnings over the years. We have not changed to better foods, fresher air, exercise and other healthier life habits. Stress, anxiety and depression are added to our other burdens. Our nerves aren't holding up as well as they should.

STEP 4: ALLERGIES AND HAY FEVER

Allergies or hay fever develop. Hay fever is a special case of allergic reaction, usually to pollens or fine particles of vegetation in the air. Allergy can be loosely defined as an abnormal, hypersensitive tissue response to pollens, dust, feathers, animal hair or dandruff, molds, drugs, chemicals, foods or other substances taken into or contacted by the body. Allergy symptoms develop when the body attempts to throw off some irritating substance.

Sinusitis or bronchitis or both may develop. (Actually, they can appear in any of the steps to asthma.)

By this time, we know we are in serious trouble. Things are getting worse, not better, despite the doctor's treatments. We may have to take allergy tests. We cut out foods to which we are allergic and we take shots to reduce the allergic response. The local druggist knows us by our first name and loves us, despite the fact that he's having trouble keeping enough antihistamines on the shelf for us.

Periods of relief are temporary, and chances are we have never thought of taking care of the bowel. Foods which cause allergic reactions have been eliminated from the diet, but we still overeat, fail to get enough exercise and perhaps even continue smoking. It all adds up to . . .

Asthma! And We Have A Bear By The Tail!

You ate it, breathed it, drank it, suppressed it into existence. "Doctor, I can't **breathe**!" "I was sure I was going to die!" "I felt like I was suffocating!" Your mistakes, your ignorance, are taking the "Breath of Life" away from you! What are you going to do?

Asthma and its brother, bronchitis, are chronic respiratory disorders which can further degenerate to emphysema and death. There are other respiratory disorders which follow the same degenerative course.

Are you ready to do whatever is necessary to get rid of it? Are you sick of being sick, ready to change your life? Sometimes we are moved more powerfully by desperation than inspiration.

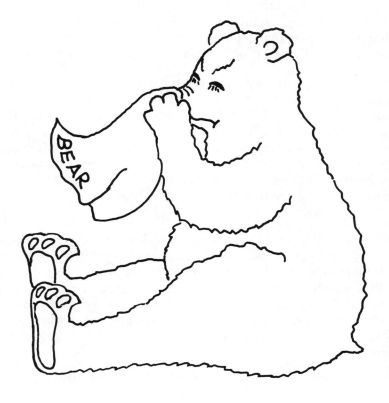

Catarrh should always be allowed to run.

19

Chapter 3. Anatomy of a Bear (Asthma)

What do we know about asthma? Well, for one thing, we know it comes from a large family. That family includes colds, influenza, inner ear infections, sinusitis, tonsillitis, bronchitis, hay fever, allergies and emphysema. These may develop in combinations in sequence, like a line of dominoes knocking each other over.

For example, you may have asthma with or without allergies. If you have allergies, the resulting irritation to the body may be expressed as itching, burning eyes; watery running nose; postnasal drip; inflammation of the bronchial tubes; itching, hive-like bumps on the skin; or any combination of these. Seasonal allergic reactions are called hay fever. Non-seasonal reactions are simply called allergies. You can have bronchial asthma, cardiac asthma and renal asthma. (We will not be discussing the latter two types in this book.)

All respiratory conditions begin with inflammation. The suffix "itis" means *inflammation*, so tonsillitis means tonsil inflammation, bronchitis means bronchial inflammation, etc. If the inflammation persists, catarrh develops and catarrhal elimination may be the first noticeable symptom that inflammation is present. The mucous membrane becomes irritated and inflamed which stimulates its glands to secrete more mucus to get rid of the source of irritation.

At this point, bacteria may come in to feed on the dead cells. Now, bacteria are always present in and around the body, but they can do no harm unless we give them an opportunity. Once a

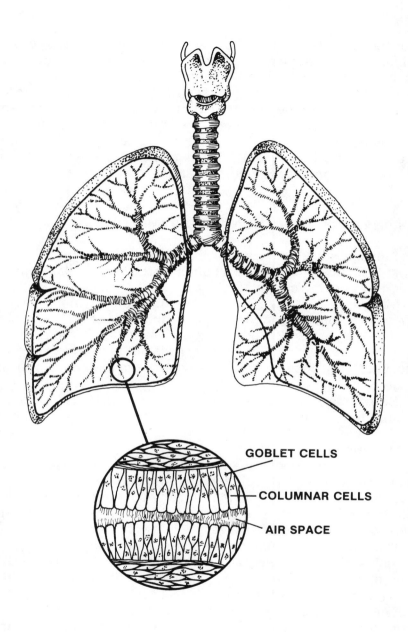

GOBLET CELLS

COLUMNAR CELLS

AIR SPACE

Inset enlargement shows swollen bronchial membrane due to inflammation, restricting air passage and making breathing difficult. Swollen bronchials can trigger asthma attacks, which represent the body's effort to throw off catarrh.

catarrhal condition has developed, bacteria may feed on and multiply in the abundant catarrhal waste, causing additional irritation to the mucus lining. This stage is called infection, and it is the stage at which antibiotics are effective, because they kill bacteria. However, they do not get at the source of the problem.

A catarrhal condition in the sinuses, nasal passages, throat or bronchials may be called a cold. If bacteria move in, infection develops, with coughing and fever almost always present. If a virus moves in, the condition is more serious and influenza appears.

RESPIRATORY CONDITIONS AND SYMPTOMS

Sinusitis starts with a stuffy nose or postnasal drip. The lower throat becomes irritated and a cough starts. Lymph glands in the neck may become congested.

Tonsillitis usually comes about from lymph system congestion, since the tonsils are lymphatic tissue. They may become infected and exude thick, yellow material. Generally, it makes no more sense to take the tonsils out to deal with chronic tonsillitis than it does to remove the nose to eliminate chronic nasal congestion.

Bronchitis is an inflammation of the bronchial tubes preceded by catarrh, coughing and colds. Bronchitis can become chronic and combines easily with hay fever, allergies, asthma and emphysema.

Allergy is an abnormal and hypersensitive response to some substance taken into or contacted by the body. It represents the body's effort to get rid of that substance. Common allergens include pollens, dust, feathers, animal hair or dandruff, molds, drugs, chemicals and certain foods.

Hay fever may include symptoms of colds, sinusitis or bronchitis since it is basically an allergy reaction to pollens or other plant substances. Often it involves inflammation of the mucus membranes of the nose, sinuses and eyes.

Emphysema develops as the walls between the alveoli of the lungs degenerate and collapse, allowing "ballooning" of many alveoli into combined air chambers. This disrupts the oxygen-carbon dioxide exchange. Too much carbon dioxide stays in the lungs after each breath to allow enough air to get into the alveoli. Shortness of breath, gasping and invalidism often result. Emphysema is fatal in many cases.

Asthma attacks represent the feeble effort of a rundown body to throw off catarrhal settlements in the lungs. Instead of being productive, such attacks increase breathing difficulty and intensify suffering, sometimes to the point of panic. In extreme asthma attacks, adrenaline injections must be given to relax and open the bronchial tubes.

CONTRIBUTING FACTORS AND CAUSES

Keep in mind that what contributes to asthma may contribute to other forms of respiratory trouble as well. We may note, also, that allergies, depending on circumstances, may be considered both a cause of tissue irritation and a result of irritation.

Asthma, hay fever and bronchitis symptoms in children may or may not be outgrown at puberty. If they are not outgrown, the progression to a chronic condition may take years.

FACTORS CONTRIBUTING TO RESPIRATORY CONDITIONS

genetic factors	lack of exercise
inherent weaknesses	stress
allergies	nervousness
climate	poor posture
chill	shallow breathing
diet	hypothyroidism
pollution	occupation
chemicals	home life
smoking	negative emotions
drugs	poor attitudes
fatigue	sluggish elimination
overexertion	blood quality
lack of rest	brain function

GENETIC FACTORS, INHERENT WEAKNESSES AND ALLERGIES

I am convinced that genetic factors play a major role in asthma and other respiratory conditions. Statistics show that most people who have allergy problems have parents or grandparents with the same problem. Hypothyroidism, which can be inherited, is associated with frequent colds, tonsillitis, sinusitis, ear and mastoid infections. Genetically-inherited bronchial weaknesses predispose many persons to respiratory problems. Iridology, the science of reading tissue conditions in the iris of the eye, demonstrates that inherent weaknesses in the lung areas are often paired with an underactive bowel (or the presence of diverticula in the colon). Toxins originating in the sluggish bowel or in bowel pockets find their way to the lung structure where they cause problems. Genetic factors may also be involved in blood chemistry, lymphatic system efficiency, posture, lung size, thoracic musculature, nervous system and glandular system which contribute to the development or aggravation of respiratory problems. Synthetic clothing can trigger allergies also.

CLIMATE, CHILL

A damp or cold climate, or a period of dampness or cold, can contribute to respiratory problems. Chronic bronchial or asthmatic patients frequently note that a breath of cold air sets off a severe coughing spell or wheezing. Of course, a sudden chill may bring on a cold or trigger an attack of bronchitis or asthma. A high, dry climate or a desert climate may be good for the person with respiratory problems. We find that climate alone cannot be blamed for asthma and related conditions, but changing to another climate may help.

DIET

The food we eat is of vital importance, not only in keeping the respiratory system healthy, but in maintaining the health and well-being of the whole body. There are four basic problems associated with the food we eat: 1) ingestion of toxic or non-nutritional substances along with our food (preservatives, artificial flavorings, colors, etc.); 2) insufficient amounts of certain nutrients, vitamins or minerals to meet metabolic needs; 3) ingestion of foods that are harmful to the body (sugar, white flour, chocolate, caffeinated drinks, etc.); and 4) excessive consumption of foods that are only good for us in moderate amounts.

Let's take the last item first. Wheat and dairy products make up an unusually high proportion of the diet in Western cultures, and they are all too frequently found to be involved in allergy problems or other catarrhal conditions. Secondly, high-protein diets, when intake of fats and carbohydrates is insufficient, can lead to hypothyroidism and consequent respiratory problems. Excess protein can't be stored in the body for later use, so digestive enzymes break it down to amino acids which the blood carries to the liver. The liver deaminates these into urea which is expelled. In other words, excess protein is treated as if it were toxic. It is detoxified and eliminated. A regular high-protein diet can clog the eliminative channels and slow down the elimination of other toxins and metabolic wastes.

Essentially, food additives do the same thing. They contribute nothing to our nutrition and they help clog the eliminative channels—the kidneys, bowel, lungs, lymphatic system and skin. Australian researchers claim that the large amounts of monosodium glutamate used in Chinese, Japanese and South Asian foods can provoke a potentially fatal asthma attack in those who are allergic to the additive.

When our diets lack certain nutrients, vitamins and chemical elements, cell starvation takes place. Depleted soils and food processing often result in devitalized foods which cannot meet the body's needs. Organs and tissues are weakened and become vulnerable to toxic accumulations and disease. If the lung structure is not fed properly, it becomes vulnerable to respiratory disease. If the thyroid doesn't receive enough iodine, the entire body is affected because the thyroid controls metabolism.

Ingestion of foods harmful to our bodies is an appalling problem in a nation as rich as the United States. A junk food diet aggravates any respiratory problem and increases catarrh production many times over the normal amount. Basically, eating junk food pollutes the body and ties up elimination channels, slowing down elimination of other toxins, drugs and wastes. Products made with white flour are often constipating. Chocolate is a common allergenic and catarrh producer. White sugar shoots up the blood sugar, draws an insulin surge from the pancreas and forces glycogen production and storage in the liver. Meanwhile, energy from white sugar is used up so rapidly that blood sugar falls and depression and fatigue set in before reserves can be released. Caffeine stimulates glycogen conversion in the liver, giving a temporary energy boost at the price of liver stress.

Many foods—or a few—may provoke a severe allergic reaction, initiating, contributing to or aggravating a bronchial or asthmatic condition. It has been suggested that not only is this reaction triggered through the bloodstream, but it may also be influenced by a reflex action in the vagus nerve, which serves both stomach and lungs and carries sensory and motor impulses. The respiratory system is very sensitive to what goes on in the digestive system. With the oxygen content of the blood down and circulating toxins up, anything put into the stomach can become a burden.

POLLUTION, CHEMICALS AND SMOKING

Air pollution is an obvious contributor to respiratory problems, as is smoking. Research has shown that it takes up to *two years longer* for foreign particles in a heavy smoker's lungs to be eliminated as compared to nonsmokers. Lead, carbon monoxide, acid fumes and many other components of polluted air are extremely toxic.

Some people are exposed to chemicals and toxic fumes more than others. Fumes may be inhaled into the lungs, or some chemicals can be absorbed through the skin. Working in paint or dye factories, photographic laboratories, pesticide factories and so on can be dangerous to the respiratory system. Even farmers these days work with chemical fertilizers, sulfur, lime, pesticides, etc.

DRUGS

Besides suppressing catarrh and contributing to the development of chronic disease, many prescription and over-the-counter drugs and remedies that relieve symptoms have undesirable side effects, long-term effects and time-bomb effects. We find that many people are allergic to penicillin, sulphonamide, bromides, aspirin and phenol preparations. Treating coughs, colds, digestive problems, nerve conditions and bowel troubles with drugs hastens chronic bronchitis and asthma.

Some drugs and chemicals are not entirely eliminated from the body but remain trapped in inherently weak organs and tissues of the body. There, they irritate the tissue and interfere with normal function, usually slowing it down.

A vicious circle develops. Accumulating toxins lead to reduced vitality. Weakened resistance invites more frequent and severe asthma attacks. The victim takes a stronger suppressant. And so the circle continues.

Drugs have their place in emergency relief of suffering, pain and life-threatening situations; but they should never be taken unless absolutely needed.

EMPHYSEMA

HEALTHY ALVEOLAR CLUSTERS

**FAT HEALTHY VEINS
FOR OXYGEN EXCHANGE**

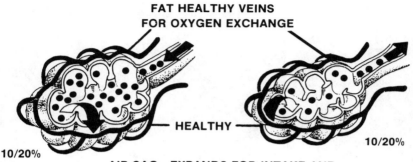

10/20%

— HEALTHY —

10/20%

**AIR SAC   EXPANDS FOR INTAKE AND
CONTRACTS FOR EXHALATION**

EMPHYSEMA—DAMAGED ALVEOLAR CLUSTERS

**THIN LIFELESS VEINS
POOR EXCHANGE**

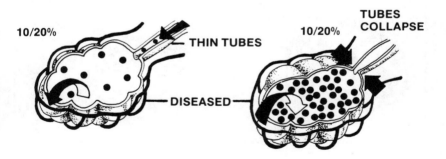

10/20%

— THIN TUBES

**TUBES
COLLAPSE**

10/20%

— DISEASED —

**AIR SAC   (BRONCHIOLES) ARE
SAGGY AND EXPEL AIR POORLY**

*In emphysema, the interior walls of alveolar clusters
have broken down, and many alveoli function together as
a single "ballooned" unit, with loss of efficiency and much
difficulty expelling carbon dioxide.*

EMPHYSEMA AND TUMORS

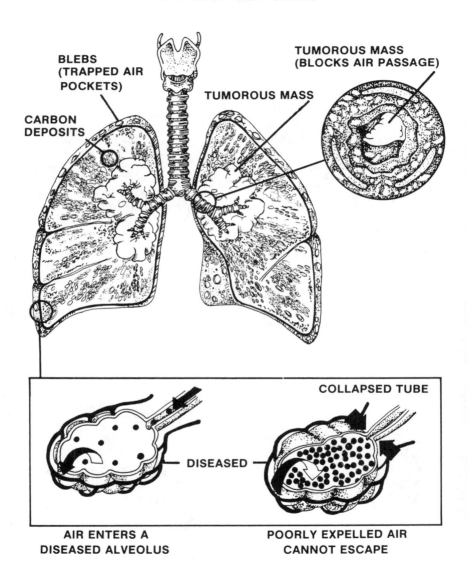

Breakdown of lung tissue due to poor nutritional lifestyle and bowel habits may lead to various degenerative conditions, emphysema and tumors being two of the most common.

FATIGUE, OVEREXERTION, REST AND LACK OF EXERCISE

It is one of the ironies of the human condition that either too much physical activity or too little can cause problems. Not surprisingly, we find that both fatigue and lack of exercise affect those who have asthma and other respiratory problems.

Overexertion, either of the mental or physical variety, leads to fatigue. In the case of someone who has asthma or bronchitis, overexertion can lead directly to paroxysms of the bronchial tubes and an attack of coughing.

With regard to those in an earlier stage of respiratory difficulties (the subacute stages), fatigue is a direct accompaniment of metabolic slow-down, a state of weakened resistance. It means the body is more vulnerable to bacterial or viral invasion, subject to toxic buildup and less able to throw off catarrh.

We must realize that exercise is necessary for proper circulation of the lymph and venous blood. Lack of exercise allows lymphatic and venous congestion to develop. The legs are the pumps that drive the venous blood back to the heart. Without good blood and lymph circulation, oxygen and nutrients are not carried to tissues that need them and toxic wastes are not carried away. Blood and lymph are the vehicles of these processes at the cellular level. The point is to exercise without overexertion.

All sick people are tired, fatigued. Being sick ties up much of the body's energy. So, those who are sick need enough rest to get well. And those who are well need enough rest to prevent them from getting sick.

Those with asthma or bronchitis often cannot rest with their bodies in a horizontal position. Their heads must be propped up high with pillows, or they must sleep in a semi-reclining position. Some can't sleep unless their feet are lower than their thighs.

STRESS, NERVOUSNESS, POSTURE AND BREATHING

Asthma is a tremendous stress-producing condition, and stress triggers release of adrenaline. During asthma attacks, this powerful hormone dilates the blood vessels and bronchial tubes. The muscles tense up and the nerves are on edge, using up extra energy and oxygen. We find that the adrenaline supply can become depleted. Adrenal exhaustion is common among those with chronic respiratory problems.

Because of constriction of breathing during an asthma attack, less oxygen is available to the brain and nervous system when it is most needed. The carbonic acid level in the blood is increased, and metabolism slows down. After an asthma attack, physical exhaustion is common.

Among those who develop asthma, poor posture and shallow breathing are frequent. If these factors aren't present to start with, they may develop along with the asthma. The forward-slumped shoulders and head reduce the chest capacity. Spinal curvature interferes with proper nerve supply. Poor posture increases the stress level and makes full, deep breathing more difficult. All these things tie in together to make life and breath difficult for the asthma patient.

HYPOTHYROIDISM

The thyroid gland, which controls the metabolic rate of the body, can become underactive due to toxic accumulations, a lack of iodine in the diet or damage to the pituitary gland in the brain. The pituitary secretes thyroid stimulating hormone.

When hypothyroidism exists, oxygenation of the body is reduced and metabolism is lowered. This affects the inherent weaknesses of the body more than other organs and tissues, and increases their vulnerability.

If the respiratory system organs and tissues are weak, an underactive thyroid can lower their resistance to colds, flu and other respiratory infections still more. Many children who suffer from frequent respiratory system problems and infections are completely freed of their condition when treated for hypothyroidism.

It is necessary to realize that standard laboratory tests such as the PBI (protein bound iodine) seldom pick up a *slightly* underactive thyroid or a condition in which one side of the thyroid is *overactive* and the other side is *underactive*.

Hypothyroidism will be discussed at greater length in a separate chapter.

OCCUPATION, HOME LIFE, EMOTIONS AND ATTITUDES

An unhappy home life or work environment can contribute to the development of asthma or to the onset of asthma attacks. An emotional component is known to be involved in asthma, but how it works is not completely known. In one study, a group of asthmatic children, removed from their home environment and away from their parents, regained their health completely within a year and had no further respiratory problems. It is worth considering whether the allergenic response may apply to relationships and events as well as to substances like pollen and cat fur.

Industrial workers may have their lungs weakened and their mucous membranes constantly irritated by the fumes they work around. The only answer to this is changing jobs.

Negative emotions such as anger, fear, envy, hate and vengefulness are destructive to the body because of the ways they affect digestion, glandular function and blood chemistry. Attitudes of self-pity, low-self esteem, "I-can't-do-it," and so forth, weaken the will to overcome and play into the hands of disease. On the other hand, asthma tends to create fatigue and depression, which open the door to psychoneuroses, poor attitudes and negative emotional responses. This chicken-and-egg cycle can be broken by a disciplined effort to change attitudes and cheer up.

THE ELIMINATIVE SYSTEM AND BLOOD QUALITY

The eliminative system is made up of the bowel, kidneys, lymphatic system, skin and lungs. All of these get rid of toxic wastes in solid, liquid or gaseous form. When any are underactive, the others have to take on the increased burden. The lungs cannot possibly be cleaned out if the eliminative channels are not working properly.

We find that metabolic wastes alone can poison the body if the eliminative organs become too congested or if their functioning is disrupted. This is autointoxication—self poisoning.

The bowel is an especially vulnerable channel. Iridology shows that inherent weaknesses in the bowel and bronchial area together are found in most asthma cases. This means they are both underactive and affecting one another. Often, bowel pockets in the ascending and descending colon indicate the presence of low-grade infections and toxic material seeping through the bowel wall into the bloodstream. This toxic material is directed to the lung structure.

The blood can only be as clean as the bowel. An underactive bowel encourages putrefaction, which affects the blood quality. Since the blood carries nutrients to the cells and brings away their waste, its role in health is critical. Toxic blood means a toxic body and a toxic brain. But even clean, healthy blood with the proper nutrients must be properly circulated to do its job, and that takes exercise. It is especially important to make sure the brain gets an adequate blood supply.

Respiration, diet and elimination all affect the acidity of the blood which must remain between a pH of 7.35 to 7.45 (slightly alkaline) to sustain health and well-being. Moreover, all three affect each other. Devitalized foods such as bread, pancakes and donuts are constipating. Shallow breathing doesn't bring in enough air to assist in full assimilation of nutrients from foods, so the excess is converted to acidic wastes. (Nor does shallow breathing allow full oxygenation of the blood.)

We have mentioned the lymphatic system before, but it is necessary to understand that it works with the bloodstream to carry off cellular wastes. (It also has some nutrient functions.) Unlike the circulatory system, the lymphatic system has no heart to pump its liquid contents. Instead, lymph is moved through its network of vessels by muscle contraction and expansion— exercise and physical activities. When the lymph system is congested in a certain area of the body, due to infection, for example, lymph nodes in the groin, armpits or sides of the neck may become swollen enough to feel with the fingertips. This means that toxic wastes are being taken in faster than they can be eliminated.

BRAIN FUNCTION

The brain is the orchestra conductor; the body with its many specialized tissues and organs is the orchestra. When brain function is slowed, the entire body is affected through the "instructions" delivered by the brain to the various organs.

Simply explained, sensory nerves bring information to the brain while motor nerves bring response instructions back to the organs and muscles. If the brain efficiency is impaired, then the quality of both input and output will be reduced.

The brain cannot function adequately without a sufficient oxygen supply and nutrients brought by clean blood. We find that asthma and even less severe respiratory problems reduce the oxygen supply and increase the toxic acid content of the blood. The levels of conscious and autonomic functioning of the brain are affected.

The vagus nerve, as we have previously stated, connects the heart, lungs and digestive system with control centers in the medulla oblongata at the base of the brainstem. (The medulla also contains reflex centers for coughing, sneezing and vomiting.)

The medulla, formed by the enlargement of the spinal cord inside the base of the skull, helps regulate respiration. The respiratory center in the medulla responds to changes in the partial pressure of oxygen dissolved in the blood plasma, not to the chemically-bound oxygen attached to the hemoglobin. (One liter of arterial blood contains 3 ml of dissolved oxygen and 197 ml of chemically-bound oxygen.) Thus, the medulla controls oxygen intake only by controlling the respiration rate. When the medulla fails to send proper nerve signals to the diaphragm and intercostal muscles, reduced breathing causes oxygen lack at the cell level.

Asthma, however, limits the rate at which breathing frequency can be increased and raises the level of carbon dioxide in the blood. Thus, the medulla oblongata is not able to control the breathing rate as well as it was designed to do. Perhaps its own level of function is lowered, adding to the overall problems created by asthma.

Considering the systematic manner in which inherent weaknesses in the body are targeted with toxic settlements, I have come to believe that a neurogenetic reflex exists between bowel, brain and inherent weaknesses in the body. Theoretically, this reflex comes into operation when toxic wastes have reached a certain level in the body. The brain, via the spinal cord and autonomic nervous system, then triggers the reflex which directs toxins originating in the bowel to the target organ. This is the first step toward chronic toxic encumbrance of tissue.

OVERVIEW

Taking a wholistic view of what asthma does to the body, we can see how many of the causal factors described in this chapter dovetail neatly into one another. To some extent, these factors

33

seem to follow one another, like dominoes lined up in a row fall one after another when one is pushed.

Genetic factors involve a special sensitivity to climate, weather and the cold. Climate and weather also affect the plant life in an area, the types of pollen and fine vegetable material that blow in the spring and fall breezes. Climate affects the mental outlook, too.

Psychological factors affect physical sensitivity, wellness, breathing and posture. Home life and type of work influence the development of psychological factors—but then so does sickness, stress, fatigue and pollution. In fact, posture influences breathing depth, nerve response, alertness and work effectiveness. On the other hand, certain types of work require that workers "hunch over" to do something.

Diet, elimination and blood quality are extremely important—but then so are brain and glandular functions. All of these things tie into the development of asthma, which makes the anatomy of this bear (asthma) seem very complex.

We do not, however, have to worry about the complexity of asthma if we keep our mind on two things. First, asthma and other respiratory conditions can be overcome. Secondly, each of the contributing causes can be changed through patient, persistent effort.

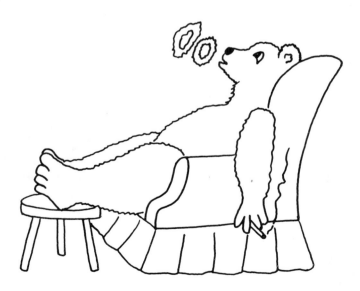

"Warning: The Surgeon General has determined that cigarette smoking is dangerous to human health (bears too!)."

Chapter 4. The Endocrine Glands and Asthma

The endocrine glands regulate important functions in the body by releasing hormones into the blood which have a significant effect on asthma and other respiratory conditions. Our emotions, metabolism and response to stress (among other things) are affected by endocrine gland function and these, in turn, have an effect on the endocrine glands. Since we know that asthma is affected by the emotions, metabolism and stress response, let's have a look at the endocrine glands and their involvement.

THYROID

The thyroid is a butterfly-shaped gland in the neck that regulates the metabolism. Now, metabolism is a term used to describe the sum of all processes in the body which build tissue, create energy and eliminate waste. That covers a lot of territory. One of the ways thyroid hormone regulates metabolism is by controlling the rate of oxygen use at the cell level. Since oxygen is necessary in most cell functions, its availability closely determines the rate of activity of cells.

Thyroid deficiency, for example, lowers the resistance of the body by reducing the rates of nutrient use, energy availability and waste elimination. This deficiency can be produced by a lack of iodine in the diet, by a toxic or inherently weak thyroid or by excessive protein in the diet. We find that an underactive thyroid affects inherent weaknesses in the body the most, further slowing or hampering an already hypoactive condition and hindering the elimination of catarrh and other wastes.

There are two types of hypothyroidism—organic and functional. Organic hypothyroidism shows up in a low fasting blood sugar test. But, functional hypothyroidism doesn't show up in most tests. According to Dr. Broda Barnes, the easiest way to test for hypothyroidism is to place a thermometer on a bedside stand at night, then take the axillary temperature in the morning before arising from bed. The thermometer is placed securely in the armpit for 10 minutes, and if the resulting temperature is below 97.8 degrees F., hypothyroidism is a likely probabililty. Women should always take this test on the second and third days of their period after menstrual flow starts, because their axillary temperature fluctuates at various times of the month.

There are children who seem to get one cold after another, often followed by ear infections, mastoiditis, sinusitis or tonsillitis. Despite antibiotics, these children continue getting sick until they are treated for hypothyroidism. Then the colds, inflammations and infections are dramatically reduced or eliminated altogether. If the hypothyroidism is not treated, these children may go on to bronchitis, asthma and emphysema.

Once a woman came to my office who had symptoms of thyroid trouble. Her doctor had ordered a PBI (protein bound iodine test) which showed her thyroid was normal, but an iridology examination of her eyes revealed an overactive left lobe of the thyroid and an underactive right lobe. (Iridology is the only science which shows imbalance in bilateral organs.) The left-side overactivity balanced out the right-side underactivity, so the lab test came out normal, completely missing the problem.

Low thyroid function allows morbid waste matter to accumulate in the body, providing an ideal environment for infections from germ life such as bacteria and viruses. Even borderline hypothyroidism lowers the resistance to the point that a little overexertion, staying up late or exposure to chill, can bring on a catarrhal condition. A history of frequent colds, flu, sinus infections and tonsillitis often leads to bronchitis and asthma later. Hypothyroidism is one of the first things that must be checked out.

We need to realize that the thyroid is regulated by the pituitary gland in the brain, and that the pituitary is regulated by the hypothalamus. The hypothalamus contains the appetite center and regulates several important body functions. Malfunction in the brain, perhaps caused by a tumor, can interfere with the release of TSH (thyroid stimulating hormone).

The hypothalamus is the part of the brain which is considered to be the basis for psychosomatic illness. Emotions affect the hypothalamus, which in turn, affects the pituitary. The thyroid is next in line. In fact, the connection between emotional upsets and thyroid malfunction is so well established that the thyroid has often been called "the emotional gland."

We also know the corticosteroids, like cortisone, reduce thyroid function.

THE ADRENALS

The adrenal glands, located atop the kidneys, produce cortisone and adrenaline. Cortisone promotes healing and is an anti-inflammatory substance manufactured by the adrenals from cholesterol. Adrenaline, also powerful, is the hormone released in "fight or flight" situations when the body needs to prepare for emergencies. It dilates the bronchial tubes, increases heart rate, raises blood pressure and energizes the body for action by converting muscle glycogen to glucose. Asthma attacks trigger adrenaline release.

Adrenaline is released in response to stress, and there are few stress provoking situations more serious than an asthma attack. The coughing, choking, suffocating feelings bringing a surge of adrenaline into the bloodstream. The adrenaline opens up the bronchial tubes and increases efficiency of blood circulation to get more oxygen to the brain and body tissues.

Over a period of time, the overused adrenal glands become unable to meet the body's demands, and adrenal exhaustion results. As a consequence, asthma attacks cause greater suffering and do more damage to the body. We find that the adrenal glands are also involved in the use of vitamin C by the body. When they are exhausted, this anti-infection vitamin is not as well utilized.

ISLETS OF LANGERHANS

The adrenal glands are not, apparently, the only glands in the body sensitive to stress. The islets of Langerhans, small clusters of cells imbedded in the pancreas, may be almost as sensitive.

These specialized groups of cells produce insulin, the substance that assists in controlling the amount of sugar that enters the blood after we eat. In diabetes, the insulin supply falls too low to keep the blood sugar at the level it should be. The blood sugar rises until the kidneys go into action, excreting the excess glucose. Otherwise, the blood would get so thick that the heart would be seriously threatened.

Our interest is further whetted when we discover that allergy symptoms and hypoglycemia symptoms can be very similar. Hypoglycemia, the opposite of diabetes, is characterized by low blood sugar, perhaps caused by insulin problems. Fatigue, tiredness, nervousness, weakness, sleeplessness and so forth are similarly found in both.

Researchers also find that asthmatics have low blood sugar and that an asthma attack can be provoked when the blood sugar drops to a certain low level. That may be the reason why asthma attacks so often come in the wee hours of the morning—when blood sugar is lowest.

I believe that continual abuse of the pancreas through consumption of excessive amounts of sugar and refined carbohydrates in the diet produce exhaustion of the islets of Langerhans, just as the adrenals become exhausted under continuing stress, anxiety, worry, fear and so forth. The shock of excess sugar may, in fact, have its main impact as a stress factor rather than a purely chemical reaction.

THE OVARIES AND TESTES

I doubt that the sex hormones have a direct effect on the respiratory system, but experience has shown that those who have a healthy sex life also tend to have a healthy bloodstream and a high count of red blood cells. We simply note that good circulation and a high blood count are necessary to adequate oxygenation of the tissues, which is inhibited in asthma cases.

SUMMARY

We need to view the relation between asthma and the endocrine glands in a wholistic perspective. That is, not only do many physiological processes and events in many parts of the body contribute to the development of asthma, but asthma affects every cell in the body. Additionally, emotions and attitudes play a role in asthma and vice versa.

Emotions, attitudes and thoughts interact with physiological processes through the hypothalamus. The hypothalamus directs the functioning of the pituitary gland, the "master gland" of the body. In turn, the pituitary directs the secretion of the other endocrine glands, including the thyroid (sometimes called the "emotional gland"), which controls the body's metabolic rate. Hypothyroidism can cause the frequent and repeated colds and flu that lead to bronchitis and asthma if not treated.

Adrenal exhaustion is associated with asthma and so is hypoglycemia, a disorder of the islets of Langerhans in insulin production.

The sex glands are only peripherally related to asthma through the functional relationship implied between a healthy sex life and a healthy bloodstream.

Perhaps the most obvious point in this chapter is that to get rid of asthma, we must take care of our endocrine system as well as the respiratory system. There is more to getting rid of asthma than meets the eye. It isn't easy to let go of a bear's tail when you've been holding on to it for some years!

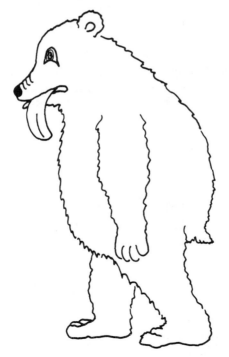

Fatigue is the starting point of every chronic disease.

Chapter 5. Health or Disease—A Way of Life

By the time of our birth, we are endowed with the physical structure that we will be living with for the rest of our lives. We come into this world with the genetic inheritance of our parents—and very little else. We have certain strengths and weaknesses in our bodies. We have gifts and talents in the latent stages, not yet brought forth. What we become depends upon the way of life we choose.

"Without good health, everything else is nothing," my mother used to tell me. Riches, intellect, great musical talent, a successful career, an industrial empire—what is any of it worth if you don't have the health to enjoy it? The answer is obvious.

THE CHOICE IS OURS

Disease, in my view, doesn't just "happen." The human body is a wonderfully made structure with a built-in natural defense system that easily disposes of most micro-organisms and other so-called causes of disease and dysfunction. We have to work hard to lower the body's resistance to the place where it is vulnerable to disease. We "earn" disease.

To get started on the path of disease, we need two foundation stones: ignorance and the drive to do things to excess. Naturally, if we weren't ignorant, we'd know better than to burn the candle at both ends. Ignorance allows us to be caught up in a temporary pleasure at the price of a later pain or ailment—the "play now pay later" philosophy.

So we eat too much, play too hard and stay up too late. We go out dancing until two in the morning, get up at six and try to do a day's work. We don't have time for a decent breakfast, so we stop off for coffee and donuts. We smoke and drink to be sociable and we worry about inflation, the world situation and whether we're going to get a job promotion. We cheat on our income taxes (just a little), lie to our friends (so we won't have to hurt their feelings) and break all ten commandments (at least in our imaginations).

Health is not the absence of disease but a way of life. We can choose the road to misery or we can choose the higher path. In over 50 years of practice, I have found there is much more to health and healing than the physical side of life. We find that the mental and spiritual aspects of life are perhaps even more important than the physical aspects—good food, exercise, fresh air, sunshine and so forth.

The consciousness of man today is far from healthy. We hear friends and acquaintances talk about their job worries, their marriage problems, financial troubles, misbehaving children and crises in other nations. Negative thoughts and emotions, researchers have shown, alter the body chemistry and open the door to disease. Hate, fear and anger can destroy anyone. We all know that chronic anxiety and worry lead to ulcers, but I believe every disease starts in the mind.

I believe in cleansing out the old to make way for the new. So, we are going to replace our bad habits with good ones. We are going to replace the experiences that tear us down with experiences that build us up.

Do you work for Ulcers, Inc.? It's time to start looking for a new job. Do your friends tell you and your spouse that your marriage is beginning to look like Custer's last stand? Call a truce and talk things over; something has to change—let it be you.

You know, we're stubborn. We think the other person ought to change. It's always the other person's fault, isn't it? No matter whose fault it is, you change first. Clean up your act, as the young people say. Then the other person will follow. He or she will change.

We are tired of being tired. We are sick of being sick. We are going to go a new way. We are going to look for the best in others instead of the worst. We are going to look for the best in ourselves, work for it and pray for it. We are going to bring in a new day.

KNOW THYSELF

"Ignorance is bliss," they say and I agree—because just down the road, the bliss always leaves and something else takes its place. Something not at all blissful. If we knew what was coming, in fact, we would have taken another road.

"Know thyself," Socrates said. It is interesting how much time we spend trying to make the other guy perfect. We need to know ourselves. We are not going to be able to get the splinter out of the other person's eye until we get the log out of our own. We need to know ourselves like we know our best friend.

Now, knowledge isn't instantaneous stuff. We aren't born with it. We gather it over the years. Nobody starts out in life with perfect judgment. We have to learn. We have to open up to guidance. How do you acquire good judgment? Through experience. How do you acquire experience? Through bad judgment. That's the way it goes.

The purpose of a good teacher is to save you some of the time, pain and disappointment that comes from learning by trial and error. Experience is a wonderful teacher, I admit, and no teacher can possibly substitute for the value of experience. But, schools don't teach us how to live a healthy life, so how are we going to find out? *Seek and ye shall find,* the Bible says. We need to be seekers. We need to become better listeners, better observers.

When we know a certain course of life is going to bring us into suffering and misery, we can choose another way. When we find a course of life that brings us satisfaction, health and joy, we know we are on the right path. Then we can turn around and help others.

There are certain things that can hinder us from finding the path of health, particularly in a chronic disease like asthma. Unforgiveness is one. Selfishness is another.

Behind unforgiveness lurk hate, anger, bitterness, resentment, jealousy, spite, rage and similar feelings singly or in combination. Behind selfishness lurk attitudes that prevent us from giving and receiving love from others.

We need to forgive for our own good. We need to love others for our own good. I know this sounds like the ultimate selfishness, but these things are true, even if they are paradoxical.

A good sense of humor is excellent for keeping our own lives in perspective. Laughter is good for the mind, body and soul and adds years to our lives. There is a healing power to laughter. Joyful anticipation is a health builder.

FAVORITE THOUGHTS

The success-minded person gets where he is going. Thoughts and intentions are mental "road maps." When you find a thought, axiom or wise saying that lifts you up, memorize it. Health, like disease, is no accident, and we need to bring our intentions, thoughts and actions into line. The mind is important. We should take as much care with what we put into our minds as what we put into our mouths.

Here are some of my favorite sayings:

> *If things aren't right, it's time for a change.*
> *Gold is valuable...Knowledge is invaluable.*
> *The only permanent thing we have in life is change. We live on memories. Start creating good ones. Harmony creates...Chaos destroys. There are no stumbling blocks in Nature which cannot be used as stepping stones.*
> *We must not let our possessions possess us.*
> *Let us nourish the roses and neglect the weeds.*
> *(These are the healing words of my mother.)*

God can only do for us what He can do through us. What we assume, we become. When we assume perfection, the Spirit goes ahead to make our way safe.

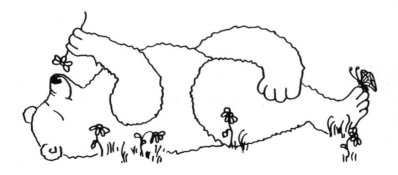

We must feel better mentally before we can feel better physically. Do more of the things you enjoy and stay away from events and people who drag you down. Get out and smell the flowers!

43

PART II. THE REVERSAL PROCESS— LETTING GO OF THE BEAR

Chapter 6. Hering's Law of Cure

Hering's law of cure states, *"All cure comes from within out, from the head down and in reverse order as the symptoms first appeared."* It is this fundamental principle, discovered by the European homeopath, Constantine Hering, that we use as the basis of our program for getting rid of any chronic condition.

How can Nature perform her duty in the body built from depleted foods and a poor way of living and thinking? There is only one answer. A change of lifestyle. Starting on the path of a better way of life, we reverse our route in search of healing crises. We have had the disease crisis. Now we must have healing crises to throw off the accumulated toxins and catarrh.

Dr. Henry Lindlahr taught me, "Give me a healing crisis and I'll cure any disease." Hippocrates said, "Give me a fever and I'll cure any disease." You have to develop a clean body; one that is strong, active and ready to go to work; a body that can rejuvenate and replace old tissue with new.

If we want to know how disease manifests in the body, we can simply reverse Hering's law: *"All disease comes from outside in, up to the head and in order as symptoms appear."* What do we take in from the outside? Devitalized food, junk food, sweets, caffeine, alcohol, tobacco smoke, pollution, noise, stress, anger, hate, fear and all degrees of toxic thinking. We take these things in and where do they go? Up to the brain. The brain knows everything that is happening in and to the body. The brain tries to direct the body to throw off what isn't good for it, but it too is affected by what is going on. Bad habits become settled in the mind. The brain becomes an accomplice to the crime of allowing certain organs and tissues to degenerate. What we take in from the outside and what goes up to the brain eventually manifests in symptoms, signals from the body that something is wrong. The original wrong, we find, was the lifestyle that led to this condition.

As we look to Hering's law of cure, we realize that we must change what is inside the body. We must get out the toxic accumulations that hinder rejuvenation of tissue. We need to take a broom into the mind to sweep out gloomy thoughts, musty memories and negative emotions, replacing them with joy thoughts, new life and positive emotions. Renewing and revitalizing the functioning of the brain further stimulates the reversal process. When the brain and body reach a certain level of strength, a healing crisis comes and the old is cast off to make way for the new. That is what we work for.

Drugs do not produce new tissues; they don't belong in the processes of regeneration and rejuvenation. Drugs control symptoms, give relief and many times cause you to relive your troubles in the future. Read from the bottle of one of the drugs so consistently used in the suppression of colds, coughs, etc., and see what it says about suppressing or relieving symptoms and controlling the cough centers in the brain. Can a drug powerful enough to alter brain center functions really be safe? What about side effects and long-term effects?

The crisis is an elimination process during which we relive old problems and troubles. The nose runs, the ears discharge, the tonsils enlarge and perhaps fever returns to burn out the metabolic waste products which were suppressed at some time in the past. There may be vomiting and diarrhea. Old aches and pains return. Psychological problems may be manifested again, but they too will be cleansed away.

When we encounter healing crises, we know Hering's law of cure is in operation and we are doing the right thing. For example, if we have asthma now, we will go back through bronchial troubles, hay fever, flus, colds and fever. If we have learned our lesson and have changed our way of life, we will never have them again.

Health is learned and earned. Health is the reward of the person who lives a better life. It is a goal to set and strive for, but we must always work for the changes our bodies need. As we start building a new body, probably eliminating catarrh or losing weight, our bowels function better and the other elimination channels improve.

When Hering's law points out that "...cure comes...from the head down," there are a number of factors we should consider. We are all born with inherent weaknesses in the body, areas that are not as strong as other areas. In one person it may be the kidneys, in another, the thyroid, in still another, the vascular system. I believe there is a neurogenetic reflex connecting brain function with that inherently weak part of the body. If the bronchial tubes are underactive and congested, brain function—possibly the medulla—is playing its part. As the conditions worsen, the blood oxygen drops and the level of toxins increases. This, too, affects the brain. Any lowering of the oxygen level of the blood lowers the efficiency of brain and nerves. This hampers the functioning of both conscious processes and autonomic processes.

Because the brain is the symphony conductor that regulates all body activities, *any condition that lowers brain function lowers the efficiency of all other physical and mental processes.* This is why it is so important to take care of the brain and nerves, no matter what else is wrong with the body. We find that it is necessary to raise the health level of the entire body to assist even one underactive organ to throw off toxic accumulations and to do that, we must not neglect the brain and nerves.

Hering's law of cure, with regard to the chronic asthmatic, is often viewed with apprehension. No one wants to retrace the suffering of those old asthma attacks. Yet, to think of a new day when there will be no more such attacks is a great consolation. And that is what we must work toward—the new day.

MEDULLA

The medulla, a portion of the brain formed by an enlargement of the spinal cord after it enters the skull, contains the respiratory, cardiac and vasomotor centers. Control over expiration and inspiration (two different centers, slightly apart), arterial and venous circulation, heart activity, blood vessel diameter, the diaphragm and oxidation of blood, lungs and tissues, is found in this part of the brain stem.

Called the "chest brain," the medulla also has reflex centers for deglutition, hiccoughing, sneezing, emesis and coughing. When the medulla is depleted, the heart, circulation and respiratory functions are affected. It is not enough to treat the lungs or bronchials during a respiratory condition. We must also take care of the medulla.

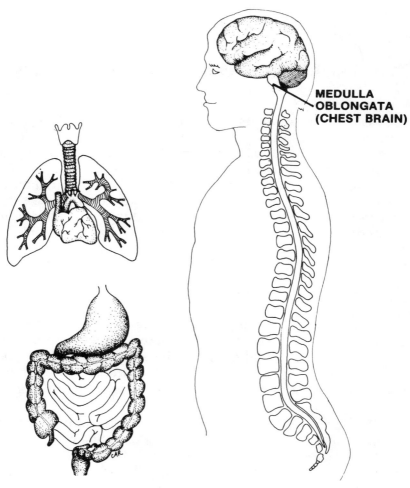

MEDULLA
OBLONGATA
(CHEST BRAIN)

The vagus nerve connects cardiovascular, respiratory and gastrointestinal systems with corresponding regulatory centers in the medulla oblongata of the brain. This is why allergens in foods can so rapidly affect the breathing, or, conversely why allergens in the air (and lungs) can affect the digestion. The heart rate is altered in either case.

Chapter 7. Detoxification and Tissue Cleansing

Asthma may be described as the body's continuing but unsuccessful effort to rid itself of catarrhal and other toxic settlements in the lungs and bronchial tubes. An asthma attack is nothing less than a weakened version of a healing crisis, and when we realize that the body is in such a debilitated condition that it can't throw off the toxic wastes which irritate and inflame the lungs and bronchial tubes, we know the body needs help. Nature is trying to bring in a healing, but it needs help. The body needs detoxification.

PRIMARY CAUSE OF RESPIRATORY CONDITIONS

The primary cause of asthma and all other respiratory conditions may be found in the eliminative system. The lungs make up one of the five eliminative channels which include the bowel, kidneys, skin and lymphatic system. Chronic lung congestion indicates that the other eliminative channels are not doing their job.

What happens when the body is picking up toxins faster than it can eliminate them? The brain, through a reflex process, directs the toxic catarrhal material to an inherently weak tissue area for storage—the lungs or bronchials in case of respiratory disease.

Excess toxic wastes build up in the body for one of two reasons. Either wastes are being produced faster than the normal capacity of all eliminative channels to get rid of them, or one or more of the eliminative channels is underactive. We need to ask why the lungs and bronchials are congested. We need to know what is going on in the other eliminative channels.

In the overwhelming majority of asthma cases, we find that the lungs, bronchi and colon are inherently weak. In many cases, the thyroid is inherently weak also. As we have noted previously, inherently weak parts of the body tend to be underactive; they do not hold nutrients or eliminate metabolic and other wastes as well as normal tissue. So, there is a tendency for the sluggish colon to throw toxic materials into the bloodstream, and there is a tendency for the lung tissue to become irritated by the excess toxins carried to it by the blood. In the process of exchanging carbon dioxide and other gaseous wastes for oxygen, lung tissue picks up enough toxic material to develop a low level inflammation.

This inflammation may be further aggravated by allergenic substances—pollens, house dust, certain foods and so forth. Catarrh is produced to protect the mucous membrane and to carry away toxic wastes, but ciliary action may not be sufficient to move it along. Instead of helping Nature get rid of the catarrh, our usual response is to suppress it, thus pushing the catarrh into "storage." We drive to the drugstore and buy a cold medication we may have seen on TV. By taking suppressant medications, we are borrowing from Peter (at a very high interest rate) to pay Paul. When Paul forecloses, we will be in deep, chronic trouble.

If the thyroid is underactive, toxins begin to accumulate in this vital gland, which cause a reduction in the metabolism of the entire body. Everything slows down. This not only increases the elimination problems of the colon and lungs, but it reduces the capacity of the rest of the body to assist and support the most seriously embattled tissue areas.

Notice that if the lungs and colon are underactive and toxic laden, the kidneys, lymphatic system and skin are the only remaining eliminative channels. Usually the lymphatic system is congested at this stage, which leaves the kidneys and skin, and they, too, have their limits.

REDUCING THE PROBLEM

The most effective immediate step that can be taken is to reduce the intake of all possible outside toxic substances. Smoking is a difficult problem to deal with, but it is one of the worst offenders. We will need to eliminate or drastically reduce the intake of wheat and milk products, citrus juices, sugar, junk foods, processed foods of most kinds. We will get into diet in a later chapter, but at this point, we need to know what to avoid.

If you know what foods and substances you are allergic to, avoid them—at least at this stage. In our chapter on diet, we will talk about a pulse test you can use for detecting allergic reactions to foods in case you don't know what you are allergic to.

Stop doing everything you know that aggravates the asthma or brings on an attack. Stay calm, avoid arguments and stress. Don't overexert yourself or get fatigued. Avoid chill or dampness.

THE PURPOSE OF DETOXIFICATION

By now you can see that the problem with asthma extends beyond the respiratory system. Many factors may be contributing to the lung and bronchial condition, and most of them involve toxic accumulations burdening the body.

The integrity of the lung and bronchial tissues cannot be restored in the presence of toxic accumulations. New cells, new tissue, will grow only as we detoxify the body, casting out the old to make way for the new. That is the purpose of detoxification.

A WHOLISTIC PERSPECTIVE

There are many approaches to detoxification which may be useful under various circumstances, but we need to approach this subject from a wholistic perspective. To clean out the lungs and bronchial tubes, we need to develop a clean bloodstream and lymphatic system. To clean up the blood and lymph, we will have to take care of the bowel.

It is not enough to take medication to "force" the body to work correctly. We need to have the right chemical balance. We need proper diet, breathing, circulation, fresh air, sunlight and rest.

We can stimulate the lymphatic drainage by taking protomorphogens or herbal teas such as blue violet. This, however, will not be sufficient to carry off toxins pouring in from a stagnant bowel holding five or six meals before elimination occurs or from one pocketed with diverticula holding trapped putrid waste.

Note from *Iridology, Vol. II*, by Dr. Jensen:

"The coming together of several unique threads of experience led me to the discovery of the neurogenetic reflex, a central principle in all healing.

"Iridology taught me why lesions in the bowel region of the iris were often 'paired' with lesions outside the autonomic nerve wreath where all other organs and tissues of the body are represented. It became evident that bowel problems were triggering reflex conditions elsewhere in the body. (Such as the respiratory system.)

"I believe the brain plays a central role in the neurogenetic reflex which links one inherent weakness (such as the bowel) with another (such as the lungs). That explains why a toxic condition in one part of the body can induce a toxic condition in another part of the body. It also explains why healing in one part of the body is followed by healing in some gland or organ remote from the first, even though the latter gland or organ is not specifically treated."

FASTING

Fasting is the most direct and efficient way of getting toxic materials out of the body. One of the better methods is to take a half glass of water every hour-and-a-half throughout the day. If it is a hot day, you may drink more, since you will be perspiring more. Avoid taking large gulps of water. The water may be cool, but not cold.

This is done along with complete rest—physical, psychological and psychic. As the body rests, it develops tone and vitality more than is possible by any other procedure. I believe fasting and rest aid healing because most energy can be focused on eliminating toxic debris rather than on operating the digestive system and the muscles of the body.

To avoid headaches from the release of toxins into the system, take daily enemas the first few days, then reduce this to every other day. If you must be physically active, do nothing to the point of tiring. Fatigue can defeat the purpose of the fast.

JUICE FASTS

I don't think any particular juice will cure anything, but I believe the rest you give your body allows it the opportunity to reverse the disease process and to recover your health. It is surprising how much energy we use up simply in preparing, eating, digesting and assimilating complex food mixtures.

The carrot juice diet involves drinking one glass of carrot juice every three hours. You can do this for ten to twenty days without problems, in most cases, or even longer. I have found that carrot juice agrees with more people than any other juice I've used.

I had one man on a carrot juice fast for a year. This man had an extreme degenerative condition of the bowel, and his doctor could do nothing for him. During the carrot juice fast, he passed mucus and catarrh continually from the bowel. Some of the accumulated toxic material was even black at times. Over the year's time, he was completely healed of his bowel condition.

THE MASTER CHLOROPHYLL FAST

A teaspoon of chlorophyll in plain water every three hours makes an excellent elimination fast which has the wonderful side benefit of building up the blood. Chlorophyll molecules are nearly identical to the hemoglobin molecules of red blood cells, and can't be made in the plant unless iron is present.

Liquid chlorophyll is usually made from alfalfa leaves, high in iron which attracts oxygen to the body. Enriching the blood with iron and oxygen during a fast helps burn off toxic waste as well as getting rid of it. I consider this the master cleansing diet for catarrh, which is eliminated most efficiently in the presence of greens.

This is an excellent three-day preparation before moving into a water or juice fast.

WATERMELON FLUSH

Eating only watermelon for three, four or five days is a wonderful diuretic, a cleansing aid for the kidneys. It helps carry off debris in the colon as well. While watermelon is classified as a food, it is so nearly liquid that it may almost be considered a juice.

GRAPE TREATMENT

Four pounds of grapes a day—Concord, Fresno Beauty, Red or Muscat grapes—are about the right amount for a grape diet. Like watermelon, grapes are mostly liquid and should be consumed at the rate of about a pound every three hours. It is important to use grapes that have seeds, since man tends to go with hybrid varieties too much.

You can eat the seeds or not, as you choose. If you eat them, chew the seeds very finely. The cream of tartar surrounding the seeds assists in eliminating catarrh. You will find that grape skins can be bitter, but this is due to a high potassium content. Potassium is a great cleanser and acid neutralizer in the body.

Especially in the beginning of the grape treatment, enemas are important to prevent toxins from accumulating. You can stay on grapes five to ten days without any supervision, but if you decide to go longer, it is best to have someone around who has had experience with the grape diet. The person should be able to handle reactions that may seem strange to you, usually variations of the healing crisis.

ONE DAY A WEEK FAST

On the one day a week fast, you can be on water, juice or fruit for the entire day—and complete rest. Many people like this one day fast. It is perfectly all right but you *must* rest to get any good out of it.

BREAKING A FAST

If you have fasted five to seven days on water, come out of it by going two days on juices, either vegetable or fruit. Drink one 8-oz glass every three hours. You have stopped taking enemas a day or two beforehand, and the idea is to prepare for regular bowel movements.

After two days on juices, start the third morning with finely-shredded carrot—steamed for one minute or wilted—to exercise and help clean out the bowel. Do this for breakfast and lunch. For the evening meal, you may have a small salad. On this same day, have a glass of juice at 10 am and at 3 pm.

The fourth day, start with fresh fruit and juice, with a snack of juice at 10 am. For lunch, have a small salad and juice, with a juice snack at 3 pm. For the evening meal you may have a salad, one cooked vegetable and juice.

On the fifth day, repeat the instructions for the fourth day, except you can have an extra vegetable at noon and again at night. You could also have an egg or a tablespoon of nut butter for the morning meal.

The next day, return to the diet recommended in the chapter on diet.

ELEVEN-DAY ELIMINATION REGIME

There are many eliminative regimes, and they all accomplish about the same results, through the fact that the body is given less food, simpler foods and simpler combinations, more watery foods—so a greater transition can take place in the cells of the body.

This Eleven-Day Elimination Regime can be used by most persons in health, and for those who want to overcome the average physical disorder. Those who are weak or feeble, however, should not follow the plan the full eleven days without supervision. Those with tuberculosis should have both supervision and assistance.

Variation, as to the length of time and the manner in which the foods are to be taken, may be adjusted to suit the history of the patient. Examples: fruits, vegetables and broths can be taken for 1 day; or 1 day of just fruit; or 1, 2 or 3 days of vegetables only.

Vegetables, taken in the form of broths, gently steamed vegetables and salads are a safer routine for the average beginner than citrus fruits.

A hot bath should be taken every night during this diet regime. Enemas may be used the first four or five days, then discontinued for natural movements. Nothing but water and fruit juices, preferably grapefruit, should be taken into the body for the first three days. Drink one glass of juice every four hours of the day. The next two days fruit only—such as grapes, melons, tomatoes, pears, peaches, plums; dried fruit such as prunes, figs, peaches, soaked overnight or baked apple.

In the six following days, breakfast should consist of citrus fruits. Between breakfast and lunch, any other kind of fruit. For lunch, have a salad of three to six vegetables and two cups of Vital Broth. Fruit juices can be taken before retiring, if wanted.

Rigid adherence to the diet is an absolute necessity for anyone attempting to regain good health. Eat plenty, but not to satiety.

VITAL BROTH RECIPE

2 cups carrot tops; 1 clove garlic; 2 cups potato peelings (1/2" thick); 2 cups beet tops; 2 cups celery tops; 3 cups celery stalk; 2 quarts distilled water; 1/2 teaspoon Savita or Vegex. Add a carrot and onion (grated or chopped) for flavor.

Ingredients should be finely chopped. Bring to a boil, slowly; simmer approximately 20 minutes. Use only the broth after straining.

WATER REMEDIES

Sitz baths are wonderful for pelvic congestion and sluggish bowels. Water should come up five inches on the body. The feet are never in the water. These baths are best taken in the evening just before bed. However, they can be taken the first thing in the morning.

The Kneipp bath is excellent for improving circulation in the legs and relieving pressure on the heart. Originally, the bath consisted of walking rapidly in knee-deep cold water for 25 or 30 feet then allowing the skin to air-dry while walking in sand or grass to stimulate the feet. Do not towel yourself dry or you defeat the purpose of the bath. Another way of doing it is to take a garden hose and run cold water first on the right foot, ankle, calf, knee and upper leg to the groin. Do the front first, then the back of the legs. Repeat for a total of three times before going to the leg leg. Again, don't dry off. Run or walk until you are dry from air alone.

THE ENEMA

I believe enemas should be used every day for a year by those who have problems with a sluggish, irregular or underactive bowel. Many ingredients can be added to enema water to increase its effectiveness in some specific manner. Coffee enemas help detoxify the liver. Flaxseed tea enemas relieve inflammation in the bowel. Over the years, I have found that the flaxseed enema is best for a sensitive bowel because it almost never irritates. Bentonite, a clay water, when added to enema water assists in absorbing and mobilizing toxins from the bowel wall. Acidophilus culture taken orally is helpful in detoxifying the bowel and in building friendly bacteria. Acidophilus implants can also be inserted rectally and left overnight.

Each of the many health professions and approaches to health care has a special value. However, no therapeutic method—no matter how sophisticated—can effectively overcome disease in a toxic-laden body. The toxins must be eliminated first. Nor can any drug-based therapy restore or rejuvenate tissue damaged in the course of chronic disease. Only nutrients from foods can do that. I believe when we work with Nature, we get the results she intends us to get. A clean body nourished by natural foods and uplifting thoughts will put anyone on the path to right living and will bring health as a natural consequence.

REVITALIZING BROTH

This broth was used during my sanitarium work with very sick people who had to be nourished back to health. It is very easy to digest.

Use 5 or 6 non-gas-forming vegetables, such as beets, carrots, potato peeling, celery, parsley, okra (if possible), chayote pear or any squash.

Do not use any of the sulfur vegetables: cabbage, cauliflower, broccoli or onions.

Add 1 cup cut-up vegetables; 1 pint water; 2 tablespoons soybean milk powder.

After either liquifying, blending or shredding vegetables, place in a pot with other ingredients and let simmer 3-5 minutes over a very low flame. This is only to break down the fiber and release enzymes.

Strain and use.

THE MINI ELIMINATION PROGRAM

In an effective bowel management program, you will need to drink at least 3 glasses of liquid before breakfast every morning.

Keep in mind that cold water will stop at the stomach, but warm or hot water will go directly to the bowel. If you want to go on an elimination program, use Veico 77 or 79 bulk and clay water. Follow directions and use it three times a day with meals over a period of thirty days. You can add more juice to your diet during that time, and you should always take juice after the bulk and clay water. If it is possible, get into some extra bowel elimination through enemas, perhaps using the clay water and coffee instead of plain water. This is a kind of elimination program you can use while working at your regular job.

THE ULTIMATE TISSUE CLEANSING REGIME

There is evidence that the sticky mucus layer lining the intestine can hold toxic material in folds or pockets for an indefinite period of time. I've seen colonics bring out grape seeds from people who hadn't eaten grapes for nine months. Similarly, popcorn kernels were expelled from one person who hadn't eaten popcorn for three years. There is, however, a more effective bowel cleansing method than colonics.

I have experienced this ultimate tissue cleansing regime and I can personally attest to its wonderful results. For those suffering with asthma, this will help more than anything I can think of.

Basically, the ultimate tissue cleansing regime aims at restoring the integrity of the bowel by removing the old toxic-laden mucus lining, increasing assimilation efficiency in the small intestine and improving the tone of the colon wall. These three improvements have important consequences. A cleaner bowel means relief for any other overloaded eliminative channels, a cleaner bloodstream and a stronger, more vital body due to improved assimilation of nutrients.

The ultimate goal is to speed up the healing crisis so that new tissue can come in to replace the old.

In my recent book *Tissue Cleansing Through Bowel Management*, I describe in detail the 7-day ultimate tissue cleansing program. Nutritional supplements, the time schedule and use of bowel cleansing equipment—the colema board—are presented in words and pictures anyone can easily follow. We will not go into them here but recommend that anyone interested further purchase a copy.

Chapter 8. Allergies, Herbal Remedies and Diet

Once the body is clean, we are ready to revitalize and rejuvenate the tissues. You can't build new tissues with drugs and you can't do it by fasting. Rebuilding calls for wholesome, nutritious foods.

Before we start out on foods, I must point out to you that food is not appropriately used by the body unless we also get enough exercise, fresh air, sunshine and rest. We are more than simply what we eat.

ALLERGIES

At some point in the reversal process, many asthma patients get rid of the majority of their allergies, but before that happens, we have some work to do to alleviate allergic reactions.

Substances carried in the air such as dust, animal hair, pollens and so forth can only be avoided in a few ways. You can put an air filter on your house or you can move to another climate. Climatology is a subject that we need to know more about. Those who have severe catarrhal conditions at sea level may obtain complete relief by moving to the mountains. In some cases, the reverse is true.

Allergies can be multitudinous, and it is hard to believe that people can be allergic to so many things. I've observed patients who were allergic to carrots. It was hard for me to believe. Carrots are such a universal food that most people can eat them with no problems at all, but we find there are exceptions.

The main allergic offenders among foods are heavy starches and milk products. Of the starches, wheat and oat products are the most frequent allergens. But, the source of the allergy is sometimes very unusual.

An allergy specialist from Chicago once sent me a patient who had developed 3,000 eye ulcers as a consequence of his allergies. They erupted after every meal. During his stay at the Ranch, he had no problems, and I thought it might be because he was eating more raw foods. When he left the Ranch, he stayed on the same diet, but the eye ulcers returned. A bit of detective work showed he was allergic to the sprays used on vegetables and to chemical fertilizers used in most commercial agriculture.

Another patient was allergic to everything but watermelon. You can't cut out everything in the diet but watermelon, so this fellow had a problem. After a fast, heavy catarrhal elimination took place, and I believe old suppressant drugs were carried out along with it. He had suppressed his catarrhal discharges with drugs for many years. He found that he could eat almost anything once he had cleaned out his body.

If you don't know what foods to which you are allergic, there is a simple test you can use called the pulse test. You will need to go on a water or juice fast for a couple of days. Then take your pulse at the wrist or throat and write it down. Do this several times to ensure accuracy. Make sure you haven't been doing vigorous physical exercise because you will need the resting pulse rate. Then, eat a single food such as a piece of broiled fish or broccoli or plums. Check your pulse every half hour or so up to three hours after you have eaten to see if the pulse rate has risen significantly. Again, make sure you aren't increasing the pulse by vigorous activity just before you take it.

Add one new food each day. Write down those you react to and those you don't. Your object is to develop a list of ten to fifteen fruits, vegetables, grains, nuts, seeds, meat and so on that do not cause allergic reactions. Later, whenever you develop a severe allergic reaction to anything, go immediately to your basic non-allergenic diet for a few days until improvement comes.

HERBAL AND FOOD REMEDIES

I am often asked if specific herbs are taken for a certain disease. They are not. Herbs are taken for a specific condition, symptom or effect. For example, a relaxant will always produce the same effect, no matter what the disease. That is what we go by.

In my lectures, I always urge practitioners to think in terms of tissue conditions, not disease. Tissue condition is more basic than the term disease, and when we have corrected the tissue condition, the disease will be taken care of.

Herbal remedies in liquid form take effect more rapidly than solid extracts or pills. For example, yarrow made into an infusion and given warm will often remove a cold overnight. We advise small doses for patients who are highstrung and nervous in temperament. The doses should be frequently administered to keep the desired result coming.

Compounds have their place, but we need to keep in mind that simply because a mixture has twenty herbs in it doesn't mean it is best for a particular condition. Often a single herb or two may be all that is needed.

ASTHMA AND BRONCHITIS REMEDIES

We believe there are a few greens to be considered for use in treating asthma. Of course, there is *chlorophyll*, which has the greatest effect, but we find *malva* to be one of the greatest ones to be used in asthma and all bronchial tube problems. *Comfrey* is another that should be used. *Comfrey* and *fenugreek*, combined, are excellent. Comfrey helps to bring down catarrh through the respiratory system and fenugreek acts as a diaphoretic, forcing out toxic materials through the skin.

Red clover is a great blood purifier used in all chronic diseases, such as asthma. *Blue violet* tea is very good to bring down catarrhal conditions from the bronchial tubes, where there may even be lumps and congestion in the glands throughout the body.

Using 8 ounces of *mullein* tea daily in asthma cases is a great help. You may not see the best results until after using it for at least one month.

Tea for relief of asthma attack. Mix equal parts of lobelia, garlic, ground ivy and euphorbia, yerba santa, blackthorn, gum plant, blue verbain and cayenne. Simmer eight tablespoons of this mixture in one quart of water for twenty minutes. Take four tablespoons as a first dose, followed by two tablespoons every half hour. When attack subsides, take four tablespoons every four hours.

Tea for bronchial asthma. Mix equal parts of sundew, thyme, fennel and silverweed. Steep one teaspoon of the mixture in one half cup of boiling water. Take one half to one cup a day, by mouthfuls.

Blue vervain a natural tranquilizer; warm tea is recommended for fevers and colds, especially for congestion in throat and chest. Aids insomnia; antiperiodic, diaphoretic, emetic, expectorant, tonic.

Garlic useful for chronic catarrh ;of stomach, intestines and chronic bronchitis. Antispasmodic, diuretic, expectorant, febrifuge, anthelmintic, cholagogue, carminative.

Yerba santa excellent expectorant; aids colds, chronic laryngitis, bronchitis, lung problems and asthma; reduces fevers; antispasmodic; tonic; expectorant; febrifuge.

Gum plant antispasmodic, expectorant, demulcent. Used in small doses helps colds, nasal congestion, bronchial irritation, spasms of whooping cough and asthma; takes up selenium from the soil; in large doses can be toxic; smaller doses may cause slowing of heartbeat.

Cayenne stimulant; toxic; digestive; sialagogue; sends blood to all parts of body.

Boneset taken warm, causes perspiration and sometimes vomiting; useful in catarrhal problems, especially flu. Mild boneset tonic: dose for drinking at room temperature: Brew a mild infusion of 1 teaspoon of leaves to 1 cup boiling water. Steep 3 to 5 minutes.

Thyme antispasmodic; carminative; diaphoretic; expectorant; sedative; anthelmintic; commonly used in throat and bronchial problems, acute bronchitis and whooping cough.

Fennel expels mucus accumulation, expectorant, antispasmodic, stimulant, stomachic, glactagogue, diuretic, carminative, aromatic.

Grindelia stimulates expectoration; antispasmodic; good for asthma, bronchial, catarrh and inflammation of bronchial mucus membranes, particularly in cases of asthma. Dose: 1/2 ounce of leaves or flowers to 1 pint water; steep for 5 to 20 minutes; take hot, 1 to 2 cups a day.

Ephedra or Mormon tea used in Chinese medicine for over 5000 years, it is a bronchodilator in the treatment of hay fever and asthma, vasoconstrictor, cardiac stimulant, major use of this herb is to relieve symptoms of bronchial asthma. Dose: prepare infusion of 1/2 ounce of the branches to 1 pint water; steep for 5 to 20 minutes; drink hot or warm; 1 to 2 cups a day.

ALFALFA TABLETS

Most asthma patients have underactive bowels, and one of the main things I emphasize in bowel health is the taking of four alfalfa tablets with each meal. Always crack them before swallowing. As far as I am concerned, this is almost a panacea. Some health professionals may think I'm going a bit overboard, but I want to tell you that alfalfa tablets provide an excellent natural fiber bulk, and by stimulating the bowel to work against the fiber, we begin to compensate for inherent weakness, by building better tone. Juice is not suitable for this purpose because pulp or bulk is necessary. Some will say that you should take the alfalfa tablets along with additional chlorophyll; I don't find this necessary, because there is chlorophyll in the alfalfa tablets as well. Chlorophyll is a great deodorizer, a great builder, a great acid neurtralizer, and one of the greatest foods for feeding acidophilus bacteria. I use alfalfa tablets mainly to get into the bowel pockets. I am sure this approach is right, because since beginning to use it, I have observed more healing signs associated with the bowel from my iridology analyses than anything else I have ever used. Of course, I'm kicking a lazy dog; I'm kicking a lazy colon.

COLDS

Whenever we feel a cold coming on, the first thing we should do is to stop eating and to start an elimination program. The latter can be done with enemas, herbs and the proper elimination foods.

It was Dr. C. H. Gesser who said that all the symptoms of a cold are typical of an acute cleansing process the symptoms of which move from within out, from the head down and whose encumbrances disappear in the reverse order in which they arose. This is Hering's law restated.

With a cold you are apt to experience a runny nose, watery eyes and sneezing. Perhaps your bronchi are congested with mucus, and you are compelled involuntarily to cough repeatedly.

When the mucus is especially tenacious and stringy, the use of Kali bichromicum taken in six-grain doses of the 4X to 6X homeopathic potencies, several times a day, is particularly effective. This may be found in a homeopathic pharmacy. For these mucus conditions, place two fresh tablespoons of each of the following herbs and add to a quart-and-a-half of cold water:

Coltsfoot
Mullein
Slippery elm flowers
Chopped licorice root

Stir the herbs into the water, bring the mixture to a boil and allow it to simmer slowly for about 5 minutes. Then strain. Drink from one-half cup to a full cup of this concoction, barely warm, every now and then throughout the day. It will make short work of your cold, and you will be surprised how effective it will be in removing mucus and phlegm from the bronchi and lungs.

Nasal catarrh can be very uncomfortable. A nasal douche can be made with 2 drops of eucalyptus oil in 4 drops of olive oil. Take this into the nose by sniffing.

COUGH REMEDIES, DEMULCENTS AND EXPECTORANTS

A strong but harmless cough syrup may be made by cutting up 6 white onions and placing them in a double boiler with a half cup of pure strained honey. Cook slowly over low heat for two hours and strain. Use warm, as often as needed.

Another effective cough syrup is made from a heaping teaspoon of linseed and a half slice of Spanish onion in two cups of water. Bring to boil, strain, add a tablespoon of honey, if desired. Take a teaspoon every hour.

If you live in an area where sagebrush or bay trees grow, pick a few fresh leaves, rub them in the hands and breathe in the powerful aroma. This soothes the nasal passages, antrums and sinuses and stimulates catarrhal elimination.

Eucalyptus leaves or peppermint tea may be boiled in a pan and inhaled to help loosen congestion and open the nasal passages and sinuses. Use a towel to make a "tent" for the head over the pan of hot, steaming liquid.

Angelica tea is good for coughs and as an expectorant. One ounce per pint of boiling water. Take two tablespoons or a small wine glass of this hot tea three times daily.

Anise seed cough syrup also stimulates perspiration and kidney function. Good for lung infections. Soothes the bronchial tubes. One part anise seeds, two parts red poppy flowers, two parts mullein; four parts each of coltsfoot leaves, licorice root and marshmallow root. Mix well and use one ounce at a time per pint boiling water; allow to cool. Take two or three tablespoons or a small wine glass full as often as desired.

Cayenne. This produces a warmth throughout the body, and we find it is a wonderful stimulant, rubefacient and tonic. It wards off the effects of exposure to dampness and cold. This is also called capsicum minimum. Capsicum is included in many of the most important herbal compounds. It is used to reduce heart pressures, especially when the digestive system is not working properly. Combined with pleurisy root, it induces perspiration.

When there are smarting and burning pains in the mucous membrane, this is an ideal remedy. The official tincture is administered in one to fifteen drops as a dose. You may take one ten-grain capsule after each meal.

Coltsfoot. A demulcent and expectorant—most valuable in bronchial troubles. Use generally with other herbs. Mixed with cayenne, it is of great value in bronchitis. One ounce of the herb should be simmered slowly in a quart of water until reduced to one pint in which either honey or licorice is dissolved. If taken in cupful doses hot, it is excellent for colds, coughs, bronchitis or asthma. One-half to one teaspoonful of the fluid extract may be taken three times daily.

Comfrey. Loosens catarrhal settlements and soothes the bowel. Excellent for colds. High in chlorophyll, iron and potassium. Comfrey-fenugreek tea is a good expectorant.

Euphorbia. Excellent for loosening tight, sticky phlegm in lungs. One-half ounce per pint of boiling water. Strain and take two tablespoons or a small wineglass. You may sweeten with honey.

Garlic is considered a natural antiseptic.

Horehound, Irish moss, linseed, licorice root, lungwort, sundew, sunflower seeds, wild cherry are good for bronchial troubles.

Onions are a good antiseptic and germicide. In the asthma diet, we should always consider using onion tea and onion syrup. Eucalyptus honey can be added to the onion syrup.

Inhaling steam from boiling coffee helps open the bronchial tubes. Hot drinks such as blackberry tea are good.

Thyme has been used for respiratory conditions for hundreds of years. You can make a powerful cough syrup by steeping or simmering wild thyme in warm water.

Herbal Combinations. For asthma relief, an effective herbal vapor inhalant can be made by boiling one ounce each of ragwort, cudweed and wormwood in a quart of water for ten minutes. Inhale steam for one-half hour three times daily.

Relief from a spasm can be obtained by adding one ounce valerian root and a quarter ounce cayenne to a pint of boiling water. Simmer five minutes, sweeten to taste with honey. Take a tablespoon, warm, every ten minutes until spasm leaves.

Here is another wonderful combination. Take one-half ounce of horehound, elecampane root, wild cherry bark, vervain, hyssop and one-quarter ounce skunk cabbage root. Boil twenty minutes in a quart and a half of water. Strain and add half a teaspoon of cayenne. Allow to cool, add two fluid ounces of acid tincture of lobelia. Take three tablespoons full or one small wine glass every three or four hours. During periods of asthma attack, keep it warmed on the stove and use as often as needed.

For inflammation of the bronchials, the following remedy has been found most helpful. Take one-half ounce of coltsfoot, comfrey root, boneset, horehound and add one-quarter ounce of elecampane root. Add to quart of boiling water, simmer twenty minutes and strain onto a teaspoon of ginger. Take two tablespoons every three hours. If catarrh removal is desired, add a fluid ounce of acid tincture of lobelia when the mixture has cooled.

We have talked so much about using drugs and their ill effects especially in producing a more chronic condition because we are not correcting a catarrhal condition in the body. There are side effects that may affect other organs in the body and give us other problems to handle. There are no side effects with herbs.

CHEMICAL BALANCE IN FOODS

From the great teacher and lecturer, V. G. Rocine, I learned the value of using foods that contained the chemical elements needed by the body. When these are lacking, cells that need them can't function. They will die if the lack persists. We will briefly cover the elements most important to the body.

Calcium, which works with magnesium to stabilize the nerves, is dissolved from the bones when the intake is not high enough. People who are bedridden or lacking in physical activity lose calcium, and this can be a problem. The astronauts on one eight-day mission lost 200 mg of calcium per day. Magnesium is a nerve relaxer. Good sources of calcium are bone meal, bran, cheese (including goat cheese), egg yolk, figs, prunes, dates, apricots, cranberries, onions, cauliflower, green vegetables, soybeans and cabbage. Magnesium is obtained from figs, whole barley, corn, yellow cornmeal, wheat bran, coconut, goat milk and egg yolk.

Fluorine. Called the "resistance" element because it is important to the body's natural immunity system. The foods in which we find the highest percentage of it are black bass, quinces, goat's milk, cow's milk and salad vegetables. Since heating releases fluorine, black bass and quinces are of little use. Goat's milk and goat's milk products are the next best. Goat's milk has ten times more fluorine than cow's milk. Warm goat's milk is excellent for the fatigued asthmatic patient with lowered digestive capacity.

Sodium. Neutralizes acids in the bowel, so it is necessary to reduce potentially toxic acidic wastes which might otherwise find their way into the blood. It also loosens catarrh for elimination. Whey, celery, seafood and green vegetables are rich in sodium.

Sodium, Iodine, Chlorine are needed to keep catarrh moving out of the body. Onions and leeks are good sources of iodine, as is Nova Scotia dulse. Onions should be eaten raw, but leeks can be made into a fine soup. Both sodium and chlorine are plentiful in vegetable juices. Chlorine is needed in the digestive system and glands. Iodine, of course, is necessary for thyroid function. Indirectly, it plays an important role in the oxygenation of the cells.

Potassium, found in all bitter-tasting vegetables, neutralizes metabolic acid wastes in muscle tissue just as sodium does in the bowel, which cuts down on catarrh production. Sodium and potassium are necessary for nerve impulse conduction across synaptic junctions.

Iron, as everyone knows, is needed by the blood to assist in attracting and carrying oxygen. "Iron-poor blood" is oxygen-poor blood, and asthma is troublesome enough without compounding the problem with lack of iron. It is found in green vegetables, liver, blackberries, black cherries, egg yolk, oysters, rice bran and whole wheat.

Silicon tones the nerves. Good nerve force is necessary to get rid of asthma. We get silicon in oat straw tea, alfalfa sprouts, rice bran, strawberries, lentils and egg yolk. Phosphorus and sulfur are also needed for good nerve and gland function. Foods containing these two elements should be eaten together. Phosphorus is in seafood, milk, egg yolk, parsnips, grains, legumes, nuts and corn. Sulfur is in egg yolk, meat, onions, leeks, garlic, cabbage, cauliflower, plums, prunes, apricots, peaches and melons.

Those with asthma need diets that include iron, sulfur, calcium, magnesium, sodium, potassium, silicon, fluorine, iodine and chlorine, plus nerve salts and nerve fats.

Foods and drinks that will counteract constipation and build the blood are needed: white clover honey, eucalyptus honey, blackberry juice, fish broth, cod liver oil, fish (the types with fins and scales), pineapple every other day.

Endive every third day. Watercress, huckleberries, mulberries, currants and currant juice, raspberry juice, figs sparingly. Leaf lettuce, boiled onions sparingly. Whey cheese occasionally. Ripe olives, pistachio nuts, almonds, carrot soup occasionally. Parsley, beets, celery soup, concentrated goat whey. Barley soup occasionally. Blueberries, elderberry juice, strawberry juice. Bitter pungent salads. Goat's milk, Norwegian whey cheese, Swiss cheese, curds, clabbered milk.

Prunes, prune juice, raspberries. Milk—but only if available fresh and foaming from the animal, not otherwise.

Eat often, not much at a time. Chew well and breathe deeply as possible. Use red pepper in the food (cayenne) to drive the blood throughout the body.

BALANCING OUR FOODS

We need to keep in mind that fruits stir up acids and catarrh in the body, but this does little good unless we have the strength to eliminate them. Otherwise, we are stirring muddy waters. Citrus fruit is the most electrically active fruit we can eat; unfortunately, it is picked green and cannot eliminate acids like vegetable juices and vegetable broths do, so we should avoid it.

The eleven-day elimination regime in the last chapter is one of the best preliminary steps to ridding the body of catarrh. The only thing stronger would be the seven-day tissue cleansing program.

We need to avoid catarrh-producing foods in our diet and substitute non-catarrh-producing foods wherever possible.

For flu—stay out of bad weather. If you get it, go to bed, keep well covered and perspire, if possible. To encourage perspiration, drink boneset tea with the juice of a lemon baked 30 minutes.

Catarrh-Producing Foods
Heavy starches: cereals (especially wheat), bread, potatoes
Dairy products: milk, cheese, butter
Citrus juices, stirs up acids
Most processed foods
Eggs (occasionally cause catarrh)

Non-Catarrh-Producing Foods
Vegetables
Most fruits
Meat; fish
Nut butters
Seeds
Milk substitutes: soy, sesame, almond, sunflower seeds
Teas

Milk Substitutes. Pasteurization is a tradeoff of benefits. We are assured of germ-free milk, but we no longer have the same food Mother Nature designed for us. Because of the substantial loss of food value due to pasteurization, I often recommend the following substitutes.

SESAME SEED MILK. 1/4 cup sesame seed to 2 cups of water, raw milk or goat milk. Place in blender and blend 1-1/2 minutes. Strain through fine wire strainer or 2-4 layers of cheesecloth. This is to remove the hulls. Add 1 tablespoon carob powder and 6-8 dates. For flavor and added nutritional value, any one of the following may be added to this drink: banana, stewed raisins, apple or cherry concentrate, date powder or grape sugar. Your own imagination or taste may dictate other combinations of fruits or juices. Whenever adding anything, run in blender again to mix. This milk may also be used as the basis for salad dressings.

I believe that Sesame Seed Milk is one of our best drinks. It is a wonderful drink for gaining weight, for lubricating the intestional tract, and its nutritional value is beyond compare, as it is high in protein and minerals. This is the seed used in the making of Tahini, a sesame seed oil dressing. This also is the seed that is used so much in Arabia and is used as a basic food in East India.

Other uses for sesame seeds. Salad dressing, added to vegetable broth, added to fruits, mixed with nutbutter of any kind, for after-school snacks, use on cereals for breakfast, add to whey drinks to adjust intestinal sluggishness; twice daily with banana to gain weight, add supplements such as flaxseed meal or rice polishings.

ALMOND NUT MILK. Use blanched or unblanched almonds. Other nuts may be used also. Soak nuts overnight in apple or pineapple juice or honey water. This softens the structure of the nut meats. Then put 3 ounces of soaked nuts in 5 ounces of water and blend for 2-2-1/2 minutes in the liquefier. Flavor with honey, any kind of fruit, concentrates of apple or cherry juices, strawberry juice, carob powder, dates or bananas. This can also be used with any of the vegetable juices.

Almond nut milk can also be used with soups and vegetarian roasts as a flavoring. Use over cereals too. Almond milk makes a very alkaline drink, high in protein and easy to assimilate and absorb.

PUMPKIN SEED or SUNFLOWER SEED MILK. (The vegetarian's best protein—sunflower seeds.) The same principle as used for making nut milks can be employed to make sunflower seed milk; i.e., soaking overnight, liquefying and flavoring with fruits and juices. Use in the diet the same way as the almond nut milk. It is best to use whole sunflower seeds and blend them yourself. However, if you do not have a liquefier, the sunflower seed meal can be used. Add seeds or nuts; not peanuts, however.

SOY MILK. Soy milk powder is found universally in health food stores. Add 4 tablespoons soy milk powder to one pint of water. Sweeten with raw sugar, honey or molasses, and add a pinch of vegetable salt. For flavor, you can add any kind of fruit, apple or cherry concentrate, carob powder, dates and bananas. You can add any other natural sweetener.

Keep in refrigerator. Use this milk in any recipe as you would regular cow's milk. It closely resembles the taste and composition of cow's milk, and will sour just as quickly. Therefore; it should not be made in large quantities.

An effective vitamin combination for hay fever is B-6, pantothenic acid and vitamin C.

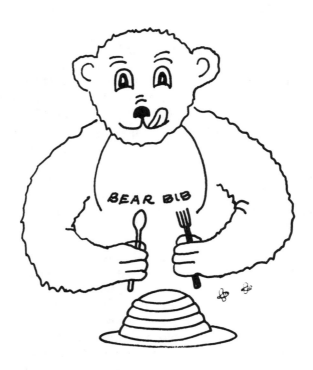

Chapter 9. Back to the Garden Foods

When the respiratory condition has begun to improve and allergies are more under control, we need to think about a regular food regimen as the next step. We are looking forward to a new day, and old food habits must give way to a new program if we are going to rebuild and rejuvenate tissue in the body. There are other aspects of life to take care of and more to learn in the following chapters, but meanwhile we must have a basic understanding of foods and diet.

From previous chapters, we can see that the kitchen is one of the keys to wellness. What we have in the pantry and how we prepare it will have much to do with how rapidly we leave old problems and troubles behind. We may have to throw away some of the foods we see in the pantry now that we know what is good for us and what isn't and replace them with vital, wholesome life-giving foods.

The best routine for daily meals should include two fruits, four to six vegetables, one protein and one starch. Drink fruit or vegetable juices between meals and eat at least two leafy green vegetables with meals. Fifty to sixty percent of the food you eat should be raw. The advantage of this diet is that you don't have to worry about getting the right amounts of vitamins, minerals or calories. It's all there.

RULES FOR THE KITCHEN AND TABLE

1 Don't fry foods or cook with heated oils.
2 Don't eat until you have a keen desire for plain foods.
3 Don't eat more than your needs.
4 Chew your food thoroughly.
5 If you aren't completely comfortable from your last meal, skip the next one.
6 Skip meals when you are in pain, emotionally upset, chilled, overheated or during acute illness.
7 Have citrus in sections only—never in juice form.
8 Avoid arguing, bickering or discussion of any unpleasant subject during mealtimes.
9 Cook at low heat using lids to prevent air from touching hot food. Stainless steel cooking utensils are best.
10 If you eat meat, have it baked, broiled or roasted. Select lean meat and avoid pork.
11 Avoid eating acid fruits like oranges and grapefruit, along with suit fruit like figs, dates and grapes or dried fruit like raisins, prunes, etc. Berries and melons should be eaten alone.

FOOD LAWS FOR WELLNESS

The 50-60% raw foods you will be eating should include fruit and vegetables (blend them if you have problems with digestion), nut milk drinks and nut butters, raw cheese and yogurt, clabbered milk, fruit and vegetable juices, sprouts, raw egg yolk, natural "milk shakes" and "smoothies" and health ice cream and sherbet.

Variety is important. Select different proteins, starches, fruit, vegetables and natural sweets from meal to meal and day to day. If six vegetables a day sounds like a lot, keep in mind that you can put four, five, six or more types of vegetables in a single salad.

In my experience, it is best to eat proteins and starches at different meals—one for lunch, the other for dinner. You can have potatoes for the starch, but they must be prepared and eaten with the skin.

Your diet shouldbe 80% ALKALINE and 20% ACID. Those with respiratory conditions often have excessively acidic bodies. The right combination of foods and cleansing the body tissue can restore the proper balance in time.

BEFORE BREAKFAST

Upon rising and one-half hour before breakfast, take any natural unsweetened fruit juice, such as grape, pineapple, prune, fig, apple or black cherry. Liquid chlorophyll can be used also— take 1 teaspoonful in a glass of water. You can have a broth and lecithin drink if you desire. Take 1 teaspoonful of vegetable broth powder and 1 tablespoon of lecithin granules and dissolve in a glass of warm water. You may have any fruit or vegetable juice. Always have liquids first thing upon rising to clean the kidneys and bladder.

Between fruit juice and breakfast, following this program: skin brushing, exercise, hiking, deep breathing or playing. Shower. Start with warm water and cool it off until your breath quickens. Never shower immediately upon rising.

BREAKFAST

Stewed fruit, one starch and health drink, or two fruits, one protein and health drink. (Starches and health drinks are listed with the lunch suggestions.) Soaked fruits, such as unsulphured apricots, prunes, figs may be used. Fruit of any kind—melon, grapes, peaches, pears, berries or baked apple, which may be sprinkled with some ground nuts or nut butter. When possible, use fruit in season.

PREPARATION HELPS

Reconstituted Dried Fruit: Cover with cold water; bring to a boil and leave to stand overnight. Raisins may just have boiled water poured over them. This kills any insects and eggs.

Whole Grain Cereal: To cook properly with as little heat as possible, use a double boiler or thermos-cook your cereal.

Supplements: (Add to cereal or fruit.) Sunflower seed meal, rice polishings, wheat germ, flaxseed meal (about a teaspoonful of each). Even a little dulse may be sprinkled over cereal with some broth powder.

10:30 AM

Vegetable broth, vegetable juice or fruit juice.

LUNCH

Raw salad, or as directed, one or two starches, as listed and a health drink. Get salad suggestions from Dr. Jensen's cookbook and food guide, *Vital Foods for Total Health.*

NOTE
If following a strict regimen, use only one of
the first 7 starches daily. Vary starches daily.

Raw salad vegetables: Tomatoes (citrus), lettuce (green, leafy type only, such as romaine), celery, cucumber, beansprouts, green peppers, avocado, parsley, watercress, endive, onion (s), cabbage (s). ((s) indicates sulphur foods.)

STARCHES. Yellow cornmeal, baked potato, baked banana (or at least dead ripe), barley (a winter food), steamed brown rice or wild rice, millet (cereal), banana squash or hubbard squash. Steel-cut oatmeal, whole wheat cereal, Dr. Jackson's meal, whole grain, Roman Meal, Shredded wheat bread (whole wheat, rye, soybean, cornbread, bran muffins, Rye Krisp, preferred).

DRINKS. Vegetable broth, soup, coffee substitute, buttermilk, raw milk, oat straw tea, alfamint tea, huckleberry tea, papaya tea or any health drink.

SALAD VEGETABLES. Use plenty of greens. Choose four or five vegetables from the following: Leaf lettuce, watercress, spinach, beet leaves, parsley, alfalfa sprouts, cabbage, young chard, herbs, any green leaves, cucumbers, beansprouts, onions, green peppers, pimentos, carrots, turnips, zucchini, asparagus, celery, okra, radishes.

3:00 PM

Health cocktail, juice or fruit.

DINNER

Raw salad, two cooked vegetables, one protein and a broth or health drink, if desired.

Cooked vegetables: Peas, artichokes, carrots, beets, turnips, spinach, beet tops, string beans, Swiss chard, eggplant, zucchini, summer squash, broccoli (s), cauliflower (s), cabbage (s), sprouts (s), onion (s) or any vegetable other than potatoes. ((s) denotes sulphur foods.)

Drinks. Vegetable broth, soup or health beverage.

PROTEINS. Once a week: Fish—use white fish, such as sole, halibut, trout or sea trout. Vegetarians—use soybeans, lima beans, cottage cheese, sunflower seeds and other seeds, also seed butters, nut butters, nut milk drinks and eggs.

Once a week: Egg omelet.

Twice a week: Cottage cheese or any cheese that breaks.

Three times a week: Meat—use only lean meat. Never use pork, fats or cured meats. Vegetarians—use meat substitutes or vegetarian proteins.

If you have a protein at this meal, health dessert is allowed, but not recommended. Never eat protein and starch together. (Notice how they are separated.)

You may exchange your noon meal for the evening meal, but follow the same regimen. It takes exercise to handle raw food, and we generally get more after our noon meal. That is why a raw salad is advised at noon. If one eats sandwiches, have vegetables at the same time.

SAMPLE BREAKFAST MENUS

Baked Apple, Persimmons,
Chopped Raw Almonds
Acidophilus Milk—Supplements
Herb Tea

Reconstituted Dried Peaches
Millet Cereal—Supplements
Alfamint Tea
Add Eggs, Cheese or Nut Butter,
if desired

Fresh Figs
Cornmeal Cereal—Supplements
Shave Grass Tea
Add Eggs or Nut Butter, if desired

SAMPLE LUNCH MENUS

Vegetable Salad with
Health Mayonnaise, if desired
Steamed Asparagus
Steamed Unpolished Rice
Vegetable Broth or Herb Tea

Salad
Baked Green Pepper stuffed with
Eggplant & Tomatoes
Baked Potato and/or Bran Muffin
Carrot Soup or Herb Tea

Raw Salad Plate with
Sour Cream Dressing
Cooked Green Beans
Cornbread and/or Baked
Hubbard Squash
Sassafras Tea

SAMPLE DINNER MENUS

Salad w/Yogurt & Lemon Dressing
Steamed Mixed Greens
Beets
Fish w/Lemon Wedges
Leek Soup

Salad
Cooked String Beans
Carrot and Cheese Loaf
Lemongrass Tea
Fresh Peach Gelatin

Diced Celery & Carrots
Steamed Spinach (cooked waterless)
Puffy Omelet
Vegetable Broth

ACID-ALKALINE FOODS

The following list of foods is from Ragnar Berg of Germany.
NON-STARCH FOODS. Alkaline: Alfalfa, asparagus, beans (wax), beet leaves, cabbage, carrots, cauliflower, chickory, corn, dandelions, endive, horseradish, kohlrabi, lettuce, okra, onions, parsley, peas (fresh), radishes, savory, sorrel, soybean (products), summer squash, turnips, artichokes, beans (string), beets (whole), broccoli, cabbage (red), carrot tops, celery knobs, coconut, cucumbers, eggplant, garlic, kale, leeks, mushrooms, olives (ripe), oysterplant, parsnips, peppers (sweet), rutabagas, sea lettuce, spinach, sprouts, Swiss chard, watercress.

PROTEINS AND FRUITS. Acid: Beef, chicken, cottage cheese, duck, fish, lamb, oysters, rabbit, turkey, veal, buttermilk, clams, crab, eggs, goose, gelatin, lobster, nuts, pork, raw sugar, turtle.

Alkaline: Honey (pure), apples, avocados, cranberries, dates, grapes, lemons, oranges, pears, pineapple, prunes, rhubarb, all berries, apricots, cantaloupes, currants, figs, grapefruit, limes, peaches, persimmons, plums, raisins, tomatoes.

STARCHY FOODS. Acid: Beans, bread, chestnuts, cornmeal, gluten flour, macaroni, millet, peanuts, peas (dried), rice (brown), Roman Meal, sauerkraut, barley, beans (white), cereals, corn, crackers, cornstarch, lentils, maize, oatmeal, peanut butter, potatoes (sweet) rice (polished), rye flour, tapioca, rye.

Alkaline: Bananas, potatoes (white), squash (hubbard), pumpkin.

Non-starchy foods mix with proteins, fruits or starches; proteins and fruits do not mix well with starchy foods.

Most people, I believe, are not allergic to the animal proteins—meat, chicken and fish; however, it is well to be aware that excessive protein in the diet may not be digested and will then be treated as toxic waste. That is, it will clog the system and become part of the problem rather than part of the solution.

In my view, a balanced food regime will include six vegetables, two fruits, one starch and one or two proteins each day. (No potatoes unless cooked in their own skins.)

Let me reemphasize that those with asthma need to avoid sugar, candy, pie, cake, pastries, sweet custards, puddings, ice cream, caffeine drinks, cold beverages, alcoholic beverages, spaghetti, macaroni, noodles, other pasta, cream sauces and gravies made with flour.

Chapter 10. Change of Life Patterns

We can't afford to lose sight of the wholistic nature of what we are aiming for in getting rid of respiratory conditions. Tissue cleansing and a healthy diet are necessary but not sufficient for our purpose. Good elimination requires exercise. Proper blood and lymph circulation simply can't take place without exercise. Shallow breathing can, in part, defeat the purpose of a good bloodstream. There are so many things all interconnected in the process of reaching specific health-related goals.

Let's see how changing some of our life patterns can contribute.

POSTURE

Posture is important for several reasons. On the negative side, a posturally imbalanced body requires more energy to maintain than a balanced one. The asthmatic tends to pick up the stooped shoulder, head-bent-forward posture simply as a response to coughing spells and periods of difficult breathing. This tendency must be fought constantly to be avoided.

Postural imbalance invites spinal misalignment and problems with the nerves.

Correct posture allows the full breathing from the diaphram that is necessary for health. By correct posture, I do not mean the head up, shoulders back, chin-in military posture which is so often associated with high chest breathing. I mean the erect posture in which the shoulders are back but relaxed with the head balanced perfectly on top of the spine.

Correct walking involves swinging the arms (which exercises the spine) and moving the feet forward with a minimum of lifting while coming down on the heel.

NERVES

As we have noticed in a previous chapter, the vagus nerve connects the bowel, stomach, heart and lungs with the medulla, the so-called "chest brain." Without proper innervation, correct breathing is impossible because the lungs cannot respond right.

Just as poor posture can interfere with good nerve supply, poor nerve supply can also influence posture. In either case, a mechanical adjustment may be required.

When we consider the chiropractic perspective, sinusitis can be caused by nerve blockages to the digestive tract that interfere with proper assimilation and elimination. Many cases of bronchial asthma involve a slight dislocation of the vertebrae in the upper dorsal region, the pathway for nerves leading to the bronchial tubes. Spinal alignment can reduce the frequency and severity of asthma attacks.

We find that interference with nerve supply can also come from drugs, from lack of biochemical elements needed by the nerves or from brain tumors.

BREATHING

Correct breathing is from the diaphragm, and the higher the chest is carried, the easier that is. Asthma comes from a Greek term meaning "to breathe hard," and we find that we must develop the chest and lungs with breathing exercises to overcome the problems resulting from asthma. Full breathing encourages wellness.

Both lungs together contain 600 million alveoli, the tiny sacs where oxygen is delivered to the blood and carbon dioxide is taken out. The total internal area of the alveoli has been estimated at 600 square feet or 25 times the area of the skin. The average adult breathes 14-20 times per minute while at rest, and resting breaths are less than a pint of air. The deepest breath we can take brings in ten times that much.

There are several "sniff breathing" exercises which will benefit the asthma patient.

Simple sniff breathing: inhale a breath in four short vigorous sniffs, exhale in one long breath. Do three times per day for five minutes for one month, then increase to four times per day for eight minutes.

Vital sniff breathing: same as previous exercise, except two short breaths are inhaled, followed by one strong exhalation. This should be done walking as well as sitting for a total of 5 minutes 3 times a day.

Whisper exercise: interlace the fingers of your two hands over your diaphragm as you sit normally in a chair. Now say, "Health for me, health for me," in a normal voice. Holding your hands in the same place, repeat that same statement in a forceful whisper. Notice the greater movement of the diaphragm and associated muscles? Good. This exercise is especially effective for those with chronic asthma. It should be performed twice each day.

Finally, here is an exercise recommended to help avoid an oncoming cold or to help in cases of catarrhal settlement. Lie on the floor, flat on your back, with legs and feet propped upon a chair seat. With a thumb, compress one side of the nose and inhale four sharp sniffs from the abdomen. Exhale through the same nostril. Take a breath through the mouth and exhale it through the other nostril, holding the first side closed. Now, inhale four sharp sniffs from the open nostril and continue these steps for five minutes.

Oxygen from breathing furnishes the heat and energy from all cellular processes. The air we exhale contains five percent less oxygen than the air we inhale, while the exhaled air contains four percent more carbon dioxide.

RUSSIAN FRAGRANCE THERAPY

I once visited a sanitarium in southeast Russia where I was introduced to what the Russians call "aroma therapy" or "fragrance therapy."

A large greenhouse was divided into smaller booths or rooms, each of which had a particular type of herb, plant or flower. There were four or five chairs in each booth.

After an interview with a staff member, a patient would be assigned to go to a room to breathe the fragrance of a single type of plant for fifteen minutes to half an hour.

Records were kept on all individuals treated at the sanitarium. Thousands of letters on file attested to the effectiveness of this therapy with various respiratory problems.

The interesting thing about this work was that some liked fragrances which others couldn't stand. It was a highly individualized process. But, people were helped by aromas they loved, whatever those were—nasturtium, peppermint, rosemary, basil, marjoram, geranium, rose, cinnamon, sage, cloves and so on.

This type of thing could be tried more extensively in this country. We use oils such as eucalyptus for aromatic inhalants in hot water, with acknowledged benefits to bronchitis patients. Anything that helps us breathe deeper may be worthwhile.

EXERCISE

Most people with respiratory conditions do not tolerate exercise well because of the limitation their condition places on rapid breathing. Nevertheless, some exercise is necessary to move the blood and lymph, to assist in the proper utilization of calcium and other nutrients and especially to get blood into and throughout the brain.

We may have to start with manipulation. We need to get to the place where we can learn to relax. Mental tensions have to go. Massage is excellent for relaxation. Any type of physical therapy which aids in relaxation could be helpful.

SLANT BOARD

Slant board exercises are the best I have found for those with severe limitations such as asthma. One of the most serious aspects of asthma is the restriction it imposes on oxygen intake and distribution. Adequate circulation to the brain is absolutely necessary before significant improvement can take place.

WARNING

Do not use the slant board if you have high blood pressure, hemorrhages, a tubercular condition, cancer in the pelvic area, appendicitis, ulcers of the stomach or colon. Pregnant women should not use the slant board. Anyone with a serious medical problem should consult a doctor before using the slant board. Those who do use it should start with simple, easy exercises and gradually take on the more difficult ones.

We find that slant board exercises are wonderful for nasal congestion, sinus troubles and other above-the-shoulder problems. Start out with 5 minutes of exercise per day. Gradually increase the time spent on the board. I recommend 3 pm and just before bed as beneficial times to do these exercises.

The majority of asthma cases are associated with inherent weakness in the bowel area, and one of the main purposes of the slant board is to bring the bowel to better tone, better condition, better function. We may have a prolapsed transverse colon, a ballooned bowel, a flaccid bowel, a lazy bowel. So we need to get to work on it.

One good starting exercise is to get a tennis ball and roll it around the abdominal area while on the slant board, with considerable hand pressure on the ball.

SUGGESTED EXERCISES ON THE SLANT BOARD

(Use Ankle Straps while doing the Following Exercises. Numbered Exercises Correspond to Illustrations)

1. Lie full length, allowing gravity to help the abdominal organs into their position. For best results, lie on board at least 10 minutes.

2. While lying flat on back, stretch the abdomen by putting arms above head. Bring arms above head 10 to 15 times; this stretches the abdominal muscles and pulls the abdomen down toward the shoulders.

3. Bring abdominal organs toward shoulders while holding breath. Move the organs back and forth by drawing them upward, contracting abdominal muscles, then allowing them to go back to a relaxed position. Do this 10 to 15 times.

4. Pat abdomen vigorously with open hands. Lean to one side then to the other, patting the stretched side. Pat 10 to 15 times on each side. Bring the body to a sitting position, using the abdominal muscles. Return to lying position. Do this 3 to 4 times, if possible. Do only if doctor orders.

HOLD ON TO THE HANDLES, FEET OUT OF STRAPS, WHILE DOING THE FOLLOWING EXERCISES:

5. Bend knees and legs at hips. While in this position: (a) turn head from side to side 5 or 6 times; (b) lift head slightly and rotate in circles 3 or 4 times.

6. Lift legs to vertical position, rotate outward in circles 8 or 10 times. Increase to 25 times after a week or two of exercising.

7. Bring legs straight up to a vertical position and lower them to the board slowly. Repeat 3 or 4 times.

8. Bicycle legs in air 15 to 25 times.

After completing the above exercises, relax and rest, letting the blood circulate in the head for 10 minutes.

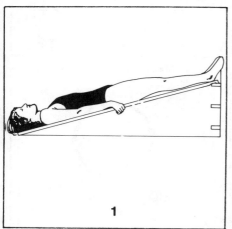

1

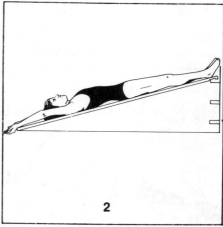

2

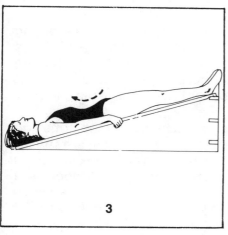

3

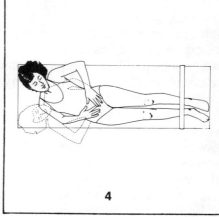

4

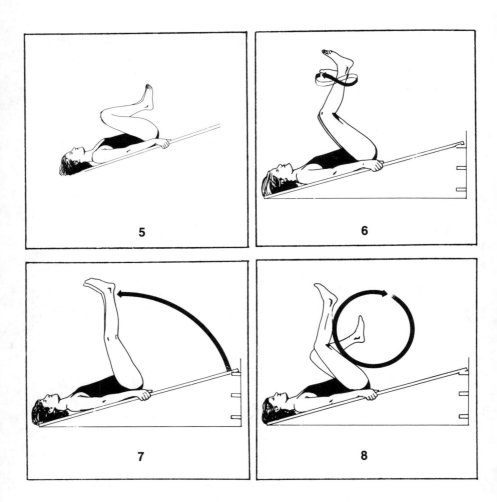

Our goals in exercising while working toward overcoming asthma are to improve the circulation, bring more oxygen into the blood, move wastes faster, develop tone in the bowel and to restore the capacity of the lungs toward normal breathing. As it becomes easier to breathe, I encourage my patients to increase the difficulty of the exercise program.

Walking is the best all-around exercise. Swing the arms and walk vigorously for at least 10 minutes each day. There are sturdy, low-built "bouncers" available on the market which look like small trampolines. You can jog in place on these machines indoors, out of the weather, while avoiding the stiff jolting to the spine, bones and internal organs that comes from jogging on pavement, asphalt or hard dirt.

BOUNCER EXERCISES

The principle of bouncer exercises is simple: we work against gravity as we bounce up, and fall with gravity as we come down, rhythmically exercising every cell in the body. Because the force of gravity operates on every cell, tissue, gland and organ in the body, the bouncer is a "whole body" exerciser.

Most people can use a bouncer, no matter how young, old, active or inactive they are. There are even beneficial exercises on it for wheelchair-confined persons. Experiments have shown that all muscles in the body are strengthened by bouncing, not just the leg muscles as we might expect, and the bowel is also toned. One man, confined to a wheelchair for nine years, was delighted at the restoration of full, healthy bowel movements within a week of exercising. The bowel, as I have often pointed out, is generally the most underactive tissue in the body and is frequently the primary source of toxic conditions in the body.

Because the bouncer is made up of a heavy-duty woven mat attached by springs to a metal frame, it has a soft "give" to it as we run, bounce or jump on it. Older people and overweight persons can use it safely and comfortably, without any jarring of the bones.

Because of individual differences in chronic conditions, we advise you to consult your physician before purchasing or using a bouncer.

The following bouncer exercises are divided into three levels of increasing difficulty. Accordingly, anyone from an invalid to an active teenager can find a level of exercise appropriate to his level of fitness and can benefit from a systematic program of bouncer exercises.

Level One Exercises. This level is for invalids, semi-invalids and those with limited movement capabilities.

The following four exercises will require a helper for the one needing the exercise. The purpose of the exercises at this level is to improve circulation of blood and lymph; stimulate and tone the bowel and other internal organs; improve appetite, digestion, assimilation and waste elimination; increase breathing rate slightly to moderately; raise the level of experienced well-being; and strengthen the body gradually, if appropriate, to do the exercises in Level Two. Also do the breathing exercises previously described.

Wear socks on the bouncer to avoid damaging mat with perspiration acids.

Exercise 1. (Do and go on to Exercise 2.) Foot bouncing. Sit on edge of bed, in chair or in wheelchair with feet near center of bouncer. Helper jogs or bounces (feet together) in time to music (or in a steady rhythm if without music). Five minutes twice a day first week, ten minutes twice a day second week, half an hour once a day third week, twenty minutes twice a day fourth week.

Exercise 2. (Do in addition to Exercise 1.) Seated bouncing. Sit close to center of bouncer as helper jogs or bounces to music. Bouncing should be gentle enough for the comfort of the seated person but vigorous enough to bounce the body. Five minutes twice a day first week, etc., as in Exercise 1. Do not do Exercise 3 until you can stand with helper holding your hand.

Exercise 3. Shuffle-bump. Stand in center of bouncer with helper holding hand if needed for balance or safety. Bounce or jog to music or in steady rhythm *without lifting feet from bouncer.* Start with 2-5 minutes 3 times a day the first week. As strength and energy increase, aim at 10 minutes each time. This exercise can also be done to revitalize the body at times of fatigue or sleepiness during the day (2 minutes).

Exercise 4. (Not to be done until strong enough to stand.) Dance movements. Warm up with Exercise 3 for 3 minutes. This exercise is fun. Select music that is both relaxing and joyful. If you have difficulty maintaining balance, you will need a helper to hold your hand while you are on the bouncer. Now, choose your own body movements to go with the music. If you are self conscious, take the bouncer to a room where you will be alone or ask others to leave for your time of exercise. Use ballet or modern dance movements, lifting the arms, arching the neck, throwing the shoulders back, bending the knees, swiveling the hips. Try a few cautious kicks, watching your balance. Let go on this one and enjoy yourself. Start with 5 minutes, increase to 10 to 15 minutes a day. Guard against overdoing at first. Many people like to keep this as a permanent part of their exercise routine.

Level Two—Strengthening. If you are able to walk, even with difficulty, you can start here. The emphasis in the following exercises is upon strengthening the body. While they are not intended to be aerobic, the exercises will quicken the breathing somewhat, so you will need to be careful to avoid overtaxing the lungs. At Level Two, it is best for those with respiratory conditions to continue doing deep breathing exercises we recommended in Level One. All body tissues and functions benefitted in Level One will be further improved here.

Many people like to bring Exercise 4 from Level One into their exercises here, and some make it their one-and-only exercise, to which I do not object. The only difference is that the music tempo should be increased, body movements should be more vigorous and the legs should be lifted higher. If you want to do this, start with 5 minutes of active, vigorous dance movements and build up to 10 to 15 minutes twice a day. Hold the abdominal muscles tight to avoid strain on the lower back. Breathe slowly, evenly, deeply in all exercises.

Exercise 5. Straight bounce. You'll be surprised and pleased at how relaxing and strengthening this simple exercise is. Keeping the feet together, bounce slowly, leaving the arms at the sides, limp and loose. Keep the abdominal muscles taut. Hold the legs relatively straight, knees slightly bent. To strengthen the legs more, bend the knees for a few bounces, then go back to the more straight-legged bounce. Start with 3 minutes, work up to 5 twice a day.

Exercise 6. Skip shuffle. With the knees bent, shuffle the right foot forward and the left foot back at the same time, then reverse. Keep this up for 3-5 minutes. Use this several times with other exercises.

Exercise 7. The swim. Using a slow, easy jog on the bouncer, do the "crawl" stroke, raising your arms, one at a time, over your head. When the left arm is as high as you can get it (reach high, stretch on each upstroke), the right arm should be down at your side. Start with 1 or 2 minutes and work up to 5 minutes.

Exercise 8. Hopscotch. Bounce first on right foot, swinging it slightly toward the center of the bouncer as you land, then on both feet, spread a foot-and-a-half apart. Do this five timies on the right foot only, then five times on the left. (It is possible to alternate right and left feet, but it is much more difficult to swing the single foot toward the center of the jogger when you alternate landing on each foot then both.

Level Three—Aerobics (for those physically active and limber).
Aerobic exercises are those that get the heart beating about double (or somewhat more) its regular pulse rate for over 10 minutes at a time with associated deep regular breathing. It may take the person coming from a severe chronic condition some time to reach this stage of exercise but it is a worthwhile goal. Those who are generally physically active, bothered only occasionally by sinusitis, hay fever, allergies, bronchitis or asthma can go directly into these exercises with the confidence that many benefits will follow.

Plan on working up to the aerobic level slowly if the exercises are difficult. Aerobic exercise strengthens the heart and builds up the lungs, chest muscles and medulla, accelerating detoxification of the body and more efficient use of nutrients. All of the bouncer exercises will bring up catarrh, but aerobic exercises bring up the most. As the lung tissues are stretched and moisturized, those with respiratory conditions will find old layers of dried catarrh are liquefied and expelled. This is as it should be, a sign of progress, the old making way for the new.

Consider that all exercises in Level Two and the dance movement exercise in Level One can be adapted to Level three simply by increasing the tempo and intensity of exercise. Always use a slow exercise for warmup and for winding down. Mix and match exercises so your total comes up to half an hour twice a day or one hour once a day.

Exercise 9. Jogging. This is a basic aerobic exercise, running in place on the bouncer. Start with a slow rhythm, swinging the arms at the sides as you would if you were running or jogging outside. Lift the knees now and then for a minute or two at a time. Work toward lifting the knees as high as the waist for 5 or 10 minutes.

Exercise 10. Criss-cross. This starts out like jumping jacks. With the legs and feet spaced a foot-and-a-half or so out on the first bounce, bring them back in a crossover "scissors" movement, alternating the right and left feet in the crossover move. Start with 2 minutes, build up to 5 minutes.

Exercise 11. Twist. With the knees bent and kept parallel, feet six inches apart, bounce with knees and legs going to the left while the upper body twists to the right, then vice versa. Do this for 2 or 3 minutes to start with and build up to 5 or 10 minutes.

Exercise 12. Combination. Start with a more vigorous version of the ski shuffle (Exercise 6), bouncing higher than required in Level Two exercises. Do this for 2 minutes, then switch to criss-cross (Exercise 10) for 2 minutes. Finish with the swim (Exercise 7) for 5 minutes. When you can run through these three exercises consecutively, do two sets of the first two before going to the swim exercise. Jog at a fast pace, lifting the knees high while doing the swimming motions with your arms.

Don't be discouraged if you can't do all the exercises in this program. The key is to do what you can do comfortably, having fun as you exercise. Older people should not try to do as much as teenagers, and those with severe respiratory problems will want to advance more slowly than those with lesser conditions. If you are following the nutritional regimen and are doing the bowel and tissue cleansing, you will speed up your overall progress by doing the exercise.

When fasting or taking juices only, do not exercise, unless to relax the body for 2 or 3 minutes with slow, easy bouncing.

Obviously, you can mix these exercises when you build up to half an hour or an hour a day. Variety is good for the body and mind.

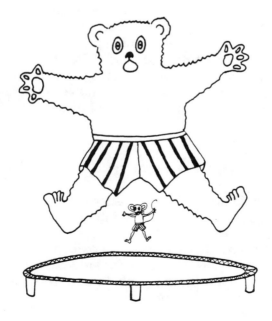

REST

Rest, of course, is just as important as exercise. Every sick person is tired, fatigued. If sleep was measured in dollars, their bank account would be way overdrawn. They need to catch up.

The asthmatic needs rest, but the problem is, it can be difficult to get. Insomnia often accompanies asthma, and lying flat on the back or stomach may make breathing very difficult. Naturally, when you can't breathe you can't sleep either.

We may need to sleep with the head propped up on a pillow or two. At this stage, we trade off postural correctness for rest. Catnaps during the day will help, if you are not working at a job.

Rest allows the metabolism of the organs to drop to a level where all available energy can be used for gaining strength and rejuvenation. Rest favors rebuilding and hastens the onset of the healing crisis we are working for.

SKIN BRUSHING

Skin cells are constantly replaced at a rapid rate, and we find that when the old, dead layer of skin cells is not continually removed, the skin cannot eliminate properly. So I recommend skin brushing as a wonderful form of "dry bathing." Get a dry vegetable bristle brush with a long handle. Never use a nylon brush.

Brush the body vigorously for five minutes each day, first thing in the morning before getting dressed. This removes the uric acid crystals, catarrh and other acid wastes that come up through the pores of the skin. This keeps the skin active, stimulates the tactile nerves and moves the blood in the small vessels near the surface of the skin.

SPIRITUAL AND MENTAL HEALTH

The wholistic view of health encompasses body, mind and spirit, and a loss or malfunction of integrity at any of these levels opens the door to dis-ease. Just as there are toxic substances at the physical level, there are also toxic spiritual and mental concepts. These need to be eliminated or changed. It is no accident, I believe that many asthma sufferers also suffer from feelings of hate, bitterness or fear. No one can get rid of asthma without giving these up.

At the spiritual level, we operate in accordance with our moral and ethical values. There are two common sources of problems at this level, and we need to know them and deal with them. First, we may have, I'm sorry to say, false religious beliefs. The belief that it is okay to cheat or steel from others is an example. Secondly, our moral values may be right, but we may be in violation of them. That is, what we do is in conflict with what we ourselves believe. Internal conflicts are caused by the latter, and external conflicts are caused by the former. Either is capable of producing the kind of stress that invites or aggravates disease.

The Golden Rule says, *"Do unto others as you would have them do unto you."* On the spiritual plane, this rule is a law. We can't break it without reaping spiritual consequences, even if we can get away with breaking it on this planet. The spiritual law says, *"As you sow, so shall you reap."* If you cheat others, you will draw much worse than that on your own head. In a sense, you can't cheat anyone else without cheating yourself more. You can't harm others without harming yourself more. You can't hate without becoming a hateful person. On the other hand, as you love others, you become a more lovable person.

Spiritual values serve as guidelines for the way our minds work. Our minds tend to measure and compare each thought, imagination, feeling or attitude against our beliefs. When our spiritual, mental and physical aspects are all in harmony, we are generally healthy and happy. When they are not, the consequences range from mild unhappiness to serious disease.

Psychosomatic disease is fact, not fiction. We find that the hypothalamus in the brain transforms thoughts and emotions into neural and hormonal reactions. The body chemistry changes. There are definite physiological reactions.

We find we cannot think sweet thoughts with a sour stomach and vice versa. Hate, bitterness, anger, resentment and fear are life threatening to those who harbor them. Many of my asthma patients have noticed that emotional upsets bring on asthma attacks. In fact, researchers have found that some types of asthma seem to be caused entirely by emotional problems and when the emotional problem is cleared up, the asthma disappears.

So what is to be done? First, realize that health is not just the absence of disease, it is a way of life. To take the higher path, you have to leave those old problems behind. Get your spiritual life straightened out. Then, begin to deal with your mental life.

Here's what to do. Go through your memory storehouse and see what needs to be forgiven and forgotten. Release all stored up resentments, ill will, vengefulness and so forth. Get these mental "toxic settlements" out of your body and mind. Stop complaining about your health and other problems, and instead find things you can praise. Look for the good in life. Avoid gossip. Stay out of situations that upset you or drag you down. Spend as much time as possible around people who love you. Avoid people who don't.

I realize that marriage can sometimes develop into a killing conflict. While I don't like to encourage divorce, we must sometimes get away from a source of aggravation to regain health. It is necessary to be honest with our marriage partners. We need to tell them we cannot tolerate certain types of emotional upset if they are unaware that their nagging complaints, accusations or critical attitudes are affecting our health. These behaviors are nothing more than bad habits. They can be changed.

Love is a healing power. Joy is a healing power. Happiness is a healing power. Arrange your spiritual and mental life so you can experience these things more and more.

Respiratory diseases often respond to soothing music and colors. The mind has nutritional needs as well as the body. Feed it well. Give it plenty of beauty. Laughter is a wonderful tonic, but be careful. Many advanced asthma cases cannot tolerate excessive hilarity or big belly laughs without triggering bronchial spasms. You can always increase the dosage as your body is able to tolerate it.

Avoid extremes. There are some things in the world that you can change and others that you cannot. It's a complete waste of energy to worry about that over which you have no power, including the future. Cultivate thankfulness. Cultivate gratitude. Stop trying to tell the other fellow how to live his life.

When we get on a good spiritual path and get rid of mental toxic wastes, we will have taken a major step toward "letting go of the bear's tail!"

CLIMATOLOGY

Although we have mentioned this before, we need to have a good understanding of it. There are major differences of climate on this planet—tropical, desert, mountain, equatorial, polar and other variations. Climate is affected by latitude, elevation, terrain and distance from the ocean. Factors such as rainfall, temperature, wind patterns, fog, snow, temperature variations, amount of sunlight and so forth, depend on these factors.

When people have lived for generations on the Norwegian seacoast, in the European alps or in the steaming jungles of tropical Africa, it is not surprising that a radical change in climate affects their health level adversely. We find that the asthmatic may need a change of climate.

Very few people live in the proper combination of higher altitude and relatively constant temperature and sunshine needed to get rid of lung catarrh. If you live in an area with cold, damp winters, try to go south for that period. The person who really wants to get well should find a way to live there three summers in a row. That may involve moving around a bit.

Keep in mind that inappropriate life patterns have contributed to the problems you now face. Changing to appropriate life patterns will not only help you let go of the bear's tail, but outrun him.

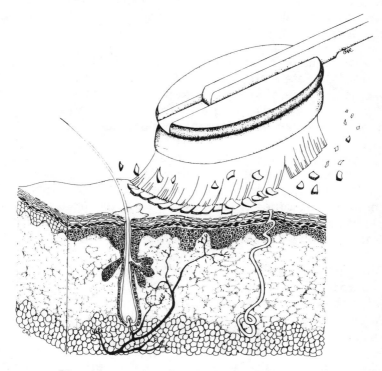

The skin, an important eliminative organ, should be brushed twice daily for 5 minutes. (Bathing or showering does not open the pores as skin brushing does.)

Chapter 11. The Healing Crisis

The healing crisis is what we are working for. It is the goal of our efforts, the object of our intentions, the pot of gold at the end of the rainbow, as far as the person with a respiratory condition is concerned. It is also one of the most miserable experiences he or she will ever have to endure.

It is worth it. Let's repeat that: *it is worth it!* I hasten to say that the truth of that statement does not rest on my opinion alone but represents the view of those brave and persistent souls who have faithfully followed the program described in the preceding chapters until their asthma completely disappeared.

The process we have described is simple but it is not easy. It was Johann Schroth, a German nature cure practitioner who said, "Without battle, no victory. Without self-denial, no satisfaction." With asthma and other chronic respiratory diseases progress is often slow and painful. A positive attitude and infinite patience are required.

Our great consolation is that we know where we are going. We have a map to get us through the rough terrain. Hering's law of cure predicts the healing crisis. *"All cure comes from within out, from the head down and in reverse order as the symptoms first appeared."*

The healing crisis is an accelerated period of symptom reversal in a person who has grown strong enough to throw off accumulated toxic wastes of the past.

RELIVING PAST SYMPTOMS

As we have said before, we may expect a series of healing crises. The way we can tell a healing crisis from a disease crisis is that it comes when we are feeling in peak condition. We are on top of the world. All chronic diseases go through regression as we build up the body's strength.

When one of my asthma or bronchitis patients has reached this point, I dread the next day. The severity and magnitude of the catarrhal elimination at times brings him right to the edge of panic, even though the patient has tried to prepare himself.

A crisis can begin small or big, mildly or violently, according to the patient's physical condition and what the body can handle.

Some crises begin with backaches, skin rashes, teeth on edge, diarrhea and joint pains. I have seen people with all these symptoms, which come on one at a time, moving from one part of the body to another.

At this time, I put patients on Potato Peeling Broth (see recipe below). This is one of the best ways I know for neutralizing extreme acids in the body and restoring potassium salts lost during severe elimination. A healing crisis usually lasts about three days but may go on for a week. It is not uncommon for emotional distress and distressing memories to come up during the healing crisis. These, too, are being eliminated. One way or another, they are connected with the development of the disease.

To have psychological debris cleared out of the mind is just as important as clearing out old catarrh from the lungs. I have had patients divulge things while in a feverish state that they denied after the crisis was over. We know there are occasionally skeletons buried in the graveyard of the subconscious that need to be brought up and properly buried. I have heard patients undergoing crises bring up memories of incidents that went back twenty or thirty years.

POTATO PEELING BROTH

Use 3 large potatoes. Cut peelings one-quarter-inch thick. Dispose of the potato center; this is the acid part of the potato. Use four carrots, eight sticks of celery and a handful of parsley. Put all of this in about a quart and a half of water. Simmer for 20 minutes. Strain and drink about one pint of this liquid daily, for 30 days.

CASE OF POTATO PARINGS

Next to Albert Schweitzer, no medical missionary enjoyed greater respect than the Labrador doctor, Sir Wilfred Grenfell. His work, too, made him keenly aware of the importance of adequate nutrition. On entering a Labrador hut, he found the father lying in a corner, extremely weak and emaciated, and the mother equally helpless, while the eldest child was barely able to get around , even occasionally to catch a fish. Dr. Grenfell was so surprised to find the two younger children running about in apparent health that he decided to learn the reason. He discovered fish and boiled potatoes were the family's chief food, and the mother not only pared the potatoes, but discarded the cooking water. But the two youngest, obeying a "hidden hunger" instinct, were surreptitiously eating the discarded peeling, raw—thus getting just enough extra nourishment to escape the deficiencies from which the rest of the family was suffering. Those extra nutrients had made such a tremendous difference!

WHAT TO DO DURING A CRISIS

During the crisis, there is no appetite. This is natural, since the body's energies are focused on something other than the need for food. At this time, the body needs water to help carry off the toxic material and plenty of rest. "Rest it out," I advise my patients, and I mean physical as well as mental.

Usually, the assistance of a doctor is not necessary during a healing crisis. The most I do is to reassure patients that everything is as it should be. Only once have I called in a surgeon to assist during a healing crisis, and that was for an extreme case. While a male patient was going through a heavy catarrhal elimination from throughout the body, he developed a swelling the size of a grapefruit in the lymphatic glands of his groin. I'm sure that his body could have taken care of this problem through the other elimination channels, but it seemed foolish to let that much toxic material circulate. It was lanced and a quart and a half of pus was drained.

Basically, what you will do during a healing crisis is to follow the natural promptings of the body, drink plenty of water and get plenty of rest.

Herb teas can be made from boneset, burdock, cascara and goldenseal. Simmer one of these herbs in water for about an hour. Strain after cooling. Drink a little at a time.

It helps to focus your mind on the fact that the healing crisis is the ultimate proof that you have changed to a right way of living. You have followed the right path or you would not have reached this goal. I don't mean to imply that you have achieved sainthood—there is always more to learn than we have time for in one lifetime, and you may go through other healing crises.

But, you are off to a flying start, well on your way to leaving that "bear" in the dust.

PART III. IRIDOLOGY

Introduction

Iridology is the science of reading tissue conditions from the iris of the eye, and through this science we can gather a great deal of insight into what is going on in the body. The iris reveals much to the trained practitioner. It reveals inflammation, where it is in the body and how serious it is. It reveals the physical constitution of the body, inherent weaknesses and the interdependence of all parts of the body upon one another.

The iris of the eye is the most complex tissue of the body meeting the outside world. It is an extension of the brain, richly endowed with nerve endings, tiny blood capillaries and other specialized tissue. Connected to every organ and tissue of the body by way of the brain and nervous system the iris is like a miniature television screen which reveals the condition of even the most remote parts of the body by way of nerve reflex changes in the iris stroma and fibers.

I have used iridology for over 50 years to assist in determining the location of abnormal tissue conditions in my patients and the stage of tissue degeneration. Iridology has been of great value to me in understanding the stages of development of all chronic diseases, including respiratory conditions. In the following chapter, I will show how useful iridology is in understanding the development and elimination of asthma and other chronic stages. For those who want to understand more about this science, I recommend my little book *Iridology Simplified*.

Chapter 12. Respiratory Problems and the Iris

Over many years, careful observations correlated with clinical evidence have allowed us to decode and learn to read the language of the iris of the eye.

To assist in reading iris signs, I have developed the following chart, based upon careful evaluation of other iridology charts made during the past 150 years by such pioneers as Ignatz Von Peczely and Nils Liljequist and upon my own research.

There are well defined pathways to health and disease which can be verified by observing the irides at intervals of time as tissue conditions are degenerating or improving.

The typical pre-asthmatic eye, for example, is mostly acidic, showing a hyperactive state of the body. The iris fibers are raised above the level of the iris stroma, demonstrating an acute condition. Every organ of the body is working to throw off catarrh. We often find inherent weaknesses in the bronchi, lungs and bowel in asthma cases. We may find a sluggish bowel or pocketed condition in the ascending or descending colon. There is a definite correlation, however, between what is going on with the bowel and what is going on in the lungs and bronchial tubes in all respiratory conditions.

We might also find a weakness in the medulla area at 11 o'clock in the right iris and 1 o'clock in the left iris showing that the "chest brain" needs special consideration.

Or we might find that the thyroid at 2:30 in the right iris and 9:30 in the left iris is: (1) overactive, (2) underactive or (3) overactive on one side, underactive on the other. If case (3) is in effect, standard laboratory analyses may well indicate normal

CHART TO IRIDOLOGY

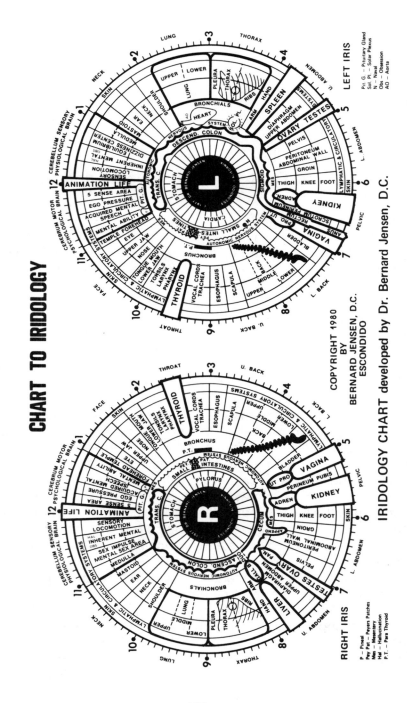

COPYRIGHT 1980
BY
BERNARD JENSEN, D.C.
ESCONDIDO

IRIDOLOGY CHART developed by Dr. Bernard Jensen, D.C.

LEFT IRIS

Pit. G. — Pituitary Gland
Sol. — Solar Plexus
N — Navel
Obs — Obsession
AO — Aorta

RIGHT IRIS

P — Pineal
Pay Pat — Payers Patches
Mes — Mesentary
Hal — Hallucination
P.T. — Para Thyroid

thyroid function. Iridology is one of the few ways of identifying this type of imbalance.

There may be other abnormalities in the iris such as nerve rings, lymph congestion, scurf rim and so forth which have some bearing upon the condition of the respiratory system.

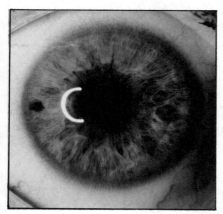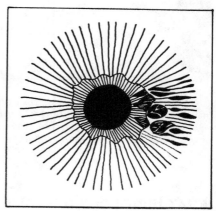

Notice in this picture that the area between 2 and 3 o'clock in the left eye is especially dark as illustrated in the schematic drawing. Check this with my iridology map chart. This darkness represents toxic settlement, underactivity, catarrhal congestion throughout the respiratory area, bronchials, lungs and pleura. This is common in all bronchial, catarrhal problems.

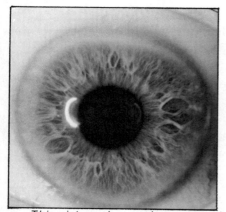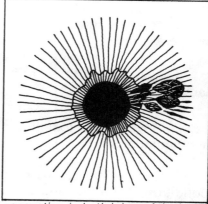

This picture shows a heavy catarrhal congestion in both lobes of the lungs represented in the left eye. The black changing to white shows new tissue taking place of the old as the result of a proper diet. This is what we look for when a patient goes through a healing.

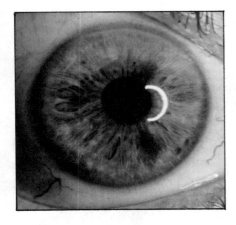
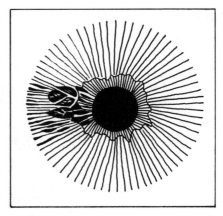

Notice the heavy dark area throughout the bronchial, lung, respiratory areas in this right eye. This darkness represents long-standing chronic catarrhal congestion that can be changed in most cases through proper nutritional procedures and bowel management.

WHAT IRIDOLOGY REVEALS

1. Reveals constitutional strength. Are we built strongly or weakly? How well does the body endure stress?

2. Reveals the health level. What is the health potential?

3. Reveals inherent strengths and weaknesses. What and where are they?

4. Reveals nutritional and chemical needs. What elements are lacking and where?

5. Reveals the location of environmentally obtained toxic accumulations.

6. Reveals the quality of nerve force in the body. What is the condition of the nervous system?

7. Reveals response to treatment; how well the body is healing itself and at what rate.

8. Reveals the acid/catarrh level in the body. Where are the accumulations?

9. Reveals the "whole" body as a unified structure. What is the "overall" health level?

10. Reveals inflammations in the body—what stage it may be in and where it is localized.

WHAT IRIDOLOGY DOES NOT REVEAL

1. Iridology does not name diseases. Often we see situations and conditions developing long before there are symptoms to which disease names are attached. Instead, we see tissue strengths and weaknesses with which we work to bring about a higher quality of health.

2. It does not reveal operations performed under anesthesia. Nerve impulses are short-circuited under these conditions.

3. It does not reveal pregnancy, because such a condition is normal for the female body.

4. It does not reveal the presence of gallstones.

5. Iridology is not a psychic analysis.

6. Iridology cannot tell specifically what accident has occurred but can see damaged tissue.

7. Iridology cannot tell specific pathology in the body. As individuals vary greatly in their ability to endure stress, what appears to be a pathology in one may not be a bother to another.

8. Iridology cannot pinpoint the location of parasites, germlife or bacterial invasions that may exist in any part of the body. It does show, however, the condition of the tissue and the development of a host situation that may allow for these things to manifest.

ABNORMAL TISSUE CONDITIONS

The four stages of abnormal tissue conditions which can be detected in the iris of the eye are acute, subacute, chronic and degenerative. Keep in mind that we do not claim to diagnose disease from the irides. Disease is generally defined in terms of a set of symptoms that can be objectively observed or measured and/or a patient's description of various subjective states such as pain, pressure, etc. We cannot determine symptoms such as fever from the iris.

Look closely at the chart titled *Pathways to Health and Disease Observed in the Iris of the Eye*. This chart clearly explains the difference between the acute, subacute, chronic and degenerative stages.

Notice in the first column how we start with colds and go down the line to coughs, bronchitis, allergies and flu. This is how the degenerative process begins. In the second column, we get into sinus trouble and hay fever. This is the subacute or underactive stage, as compared to the acute or overactive stage in column one. When we suppress the catarrhal runoff indicated in stage one, we drive the problem deeper into the tissues and begin to compromise tissue integrity. Metabolic processes are forced to slow down. Column three, the chronic stage, shows pneumonia and asthma. Column four, the degenerative stage, indicates that emphysema and other extreme conditions have developed.

We can't tell from the iris precisely when colds have shifted into bronchitis or when hay fever has developed into asthma. But we can tell whether the condition is getting better or worse. Best of all, we know from the iris what we need to do.

Iridology and nutrition work hand in hand. We can design a diet program intended to cleanse the bowel, improve the bloodstream and strengthen the body. We can see when our program is working by noticing whether the irides are growing lighter. If they are, we are on the right track.

HERING'S LAW AND THE IRIS

As we follow Hering's law of cure and the reversal process in the iris of the eye, we will find the iris growing lighter in color. If we carefully inspect the holes or lesions, we will see that fine white filaments called healing lines are coming in. This means our program is working. If that were all iridology could tell us, it would still be a wonderful analytic tool.

When the body is approaching a healing crisis, the iris fibers move into the acute stage. We're not talking about only the iris fibers of the respiratory system and the bowel but all iris fibers. A healing crisis involves all the organs and systems of the body, which means that tissues have grown strong enough to function in a hyperactive state long enough for a powerful catarrhal elimination.

PATHWAYS TO HEALTH AND DISEASE OBSERVED IN THE IRIS OF THE EYE

ACCORDING TO HERING'S LAW OF CURE: "All cure starts from within out, from the head down and in the reverse order as the symptoms have appeared."

This chart illustrates the correlation between the natural light of the iris and good health versus the darkness of the iris in proportion to the degree of degeneration in the body.

BY BERNARD JENSEN, DC, ND

INDICATION IN IRIS	• WHITE •	• LIGHT GRAY •	• DARK GRAY •	• BLACK •
STAGE	ACUTE	SUBACUTE	CHRONIC	DEGENERATIVE
ASSOCIATED SIGNS	ELEVATED	JUST BELOW SURFACE	WELL BELOW SURFACE	COMPLETELY RECESSED
SYMPTOMS IN BODY	Inflammation. Pain. Sensitivity. Fever. Discharge. High Activity	Toxic Absorption. Low Metabolism. Weak Condition. Less Pain	Low Metabolic Activity. Toxic buildup. Lack of Vitality	No Sensation. Circulation. Tissue Decay
CATARRH-ACID LEVEL (TOXIC ACCUMULATION)	Poor living habits contribute to the infiltration of catarrhal buildup and the beginning of toxic settlements	Junk food, devitalized foods poor dietary habits, polluted environment - toxic settlements begin to build	Heavy accumulation interfere with cellular activity	Limit of toxic settlement body can tolerate, breakdown of life-giving activity. Vital force at lowest ebb.

DEGENERATIVE PROCESSES:
ARTHRITIS
EMPHYSEMA
MALIGNANCY

FACTORS THAT UNDERMINE HEALTH & VITALITY:
HEREDITARY FACTORS
CHILDHOOD FACTORS

A healing crisis develops on the path at approximately the same point as the original ailment.

Healing Crisis and Reversal Process as shown in the color of the iris.

(WHERE ARE YOU ALONG THIS PATH?)

WE DON'T CATCH DISEASES, WE CREATE THEM BY BREAKING DOWN THE NATURAL DEFENSES ACCORDING TO THE WAY WE EAT, DRINK, THINK AND LIVE.

TISSUE INTEGRITY OR HEALTH LEVEL — HIGH ... LOW

TOWARD ILLNESS AND DISEASE

TOWARD HEALING REJUVENATION

HAY FEVER
SINUS — Discharges from nose eyes.
Suppression: Sprays. vapors synthetic chemicals
ALLERGIES
FLU
BRONCHITIS
COUGHS
COLDS
Suppression: Coal tar drugs, motrum, aspirin, etc.
PNEUMONIA
ASTHMA
Suppression: analgesics, acids, Drugs tranquilizers
Healing: Tissue cleansing, toxic elimination, correct diet
Suppression: Cortisone chemotherapy, radiation, heavy drugs

TUMORS
ARTHRITIS
GANGRENE
EMPHYSEMA
HARDENING of ARTERIES
MALIGNANCY

(BIRTH) — 2 Years — 11 Years — 28 Years — Any age — (DEATH)

CHART TO IRIDOLOGY

RIGHT IRIS   LEFT IRIS

(1) FROM THE HEAD DOWN
(2) FROM THE INSIDE OUT
(3) IN THE REVERSE ORDER

FIRST TO HEAL
SECOND TO HEAL
THIRD TO HEAL
FOURTH TO HEAL

THE REVERSAL PATH TO A HIGHER HEALTH LEVEL
FUNDAMENTALS FOR STARTING

This chart illustrates Hering's law of cure by showing the paths that lead to disease and revitalization, as they are one and the same. This concept is vitally important to the understanding of the "reversal process" and the amazing phenomena of the healing body as it responds to natural, pure and whole remedies. Full color chart measuring 11 by 17 inches is available from the publisher, see last page for address.

The main problem may be in the lungs and bronchial tubes, but it takes the whole body to deal with it. This means we have to do more than simply try to clean up and rejuvenate the lung areas to successfully get rid of respiratory disease. The iris teaches us that we must cleanse and build up the entire body to assist one area in chronic condition to expel toxic settlements.

We don't simply "catch" asthma. We earn it; we work for it. We eat and drink our way to asthma. We invite it by a lack of proper spiritual values, by showing the wrong attitude, by thinking the wrong thoughts. Our job, environment, financial condition and marriage or our attitude toward any of these may have contributed to the emergence of asthma.

There is a life story, a history, in each iris. Inherent weaknesses may be genetically determined, but we can avoid running the body down to the point where those weaknesses become cesspools of toxic waste storage. Everything in the body needs to flow or change. We don't want anything to be stopped which is meant by nature to move in (oxygen, water, nutrients) or move out (wastes).

Portions of the iris change from white to gray to dark gray. The movement from light to darkness means trouble. Try to remember that. On the other hand, the shift from darkness to light means good news.

When the eye finally turns white again, that is the best news of all. That means a healing crisis is coming—and soon.

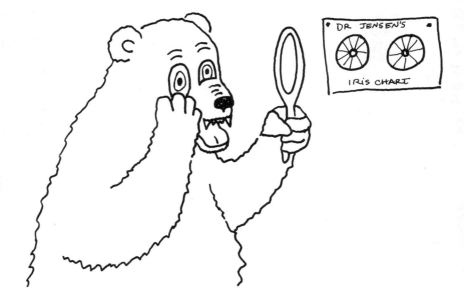

PART IV. ASTHMA CASE HISTORIES

The most reliable evidence, whether in a court of law or a scientific laboratory, is called "first-hand" evidence. "This is what happened to me," says someone. "I saw it with my own eyes," or "I heard it with my own ears." We are always hearing secondhand about a great cure or miraculous recovery that happened to someone else. But when we ourselves go through an experience, we know what happened in such an intimate, personal way that no one can shake us or cause us to doubt.

Melvina Dye and a Patient from Maryland have gone through my program. Their personal testimonies speak much more powerfully than anything I can say about the effectiveness of nutrition and tissue cleansing in reversing the symptoms of chronic asthma. Everyone is looking for a good doctor, but I look for good patients—like Melvina Dye and the Patient from Maryland—who faithfully go through the program, following directions and doing the work they need to do.

These two wonderful ladies deserve the health level they are now enjoying. They have certainly earned it by their patience, courage and willingness to change to a new path and leave the old life behind.

Following the testimonies of these remarkable ladies, two short interviews are presented which give further insight into the effectiveness of the program described in this book.

Chapter 13. Personal Testimonies

Melvina Dye

In September of 1973, I had a physical examination and was told that I was in good health. One month later I could scarcely walk across the room—no energy and great difficulty in breathing. I returned to the doctor, and he told me I had asthma. He suggested I think about retiring and perhaps going south for the winter. I did this but spent the time, continually it seemed, in the hospital or the emergency room fighting for my breath. Little did I know this would turn into weeks, then to months, and then to years before I would find the right path to follow.

Throughout my life, I had always thought I was well-grounded in my faith in God, but at that time, I found myself confronted with problems testing my faith to the limit—six great bereavements, my health failing and vital forces being depleted.

Three years passed and my health seemed to be going downhill daily. At this point, I was taking antibiotics and a cortisone drug about every three weeks. I would no sooner complete one series than it would be necessary to start another round. I believe the drugs also suppressed my condition and created a more chronic condition. Now I know never to stop catarrhal, phlegm or mucus discharges. I realize it is necessary to give my body its will to cleanse and purify itself.

It was almost three years later on May 28, 1976, that I stood in front of the mirror and took a good long look at myself. I knew I would not be here long if help did not come soon. Then as I walked into the kitchen, I saw Dr. Bernard Jensen's cookbook, *Vital Foods for Total Health*. I picked it up and on the very last page, I read about the "Place to regain health" and about the treatment in his clinic of various catarrhal disturbances, such as bronchitis, asthma, hay fever and so forth. This is what I wanted to do—go to Hidden Valley Health Ranch in Escondido, California.

Sometimes truth is stranger than fiction, because the next morning, a very dear friend called and asked if I would go with her "to see Dr. Bernard Jensen in Escondido, California!" I was speechless for a moment, but when I found my voice, we called and made arrangements for a three-week stay at Dr. Jensen's Ranch.

Two weeks later we arrived at the Ranch, and the next morning, I had my first visit with Dr. Jensen. He took my blood pressure, looked at my hands and examined both irides. Then he looked at me and said, "My dear, I would rather go out the back door than treat asthma patients!"

He asked me where I had been all this time, and I said that I didn't know about his work. I heard him telling me not only that I had problems in the lung area but that I had one weak kidney, three pockets on one side of the large colon and four pockets on the other side of the large colon, hardening of the arteries in the legs, exhausted adrenal glands, inactive pancreas, a lack of hydrochloric acid in the stomach and an inability to assimilate food. Nerve rings showed that I had carried too much of a load in the past. I also showed a heart problem, brain anemia and some arthritis in the shoulders, an all-acid body, and a scurf rim showing the underactivity of the tissues involved, mainly the skin and circulatory systems.

Tears of joy started streaming down my face...I recognized all the different things he was bringing out in his analysis...I knew within me that at last I had been led to the right doctor!

Instead of staying three weeks, I stayed three months. This was the greatest decision of my life. This reeducation experience literally turned my life around—moving lifeward instead of deathward.

When I came into this world, I was sick a whole year. Then when I was six or seven, I had double pneumonia and was given up to die. I had pneumonia a couple of other times in my life. Possibly this inherent weakness in my background came through the family, as my maternal grandmother had lung problems or asthma and my father had hay fever.

During my teen years, I was under great mental stress and later during a 44-year working period, all of the four positions I held carried great responsibilities, long hours and considerable pressure.

My marriage of 45 years presented many challenges. During the 32nd year, my husband underwent five eye surgeries in four months. Eight years later he had two strokes and we finally learned he had a very serious lung condition before his passing.

Like many others, my life had been one of overcoming obstacles, but I found asthma to be something that stumped all experts. I had to change if I wanted to breathe.

During my three-month stay at the Ranch, I attended all lectures, summer classes and iridology seminars. I made up my mind to be an apt student and learn this new way that was offering the possibility of relief. There were daily activities of exercise and walking at the Ranch, and I wanted to participate as much as possible, but I had no energy. I barely made it to meals.

I reported frequently to Dr. Jensen. After a few days of not much progress, I was given raw goat milk twice a day. I became stronger, had more vitality and gained some weight. Also, my body was beginning to respond to the raw salads and good food. Every day I had six vegetables, two fruits, one protein and one starch. Sixty percent of my food was raw.

Eliminating junk foods is not always pleasant, as the toxic materials begin to work out of the body. I experienced several healing crises and each time became stronger. My body was exchanging the lower for the higher values. I learned it would take from one to two years or more to renew the cells and tissues as the body must have all the chemicals and minerals as nature provides during the four seasons.

One of the best stories I learned at the Ranch was about variety. If you will get a variety and have a rainbow salad with all the colors which represent all the minerals, all the vitamins, you will not make mistakes. When you have a rainbow salad, you have vitamins A, B, E and C, silicon, calcium, sodium, and so forth. It is necessary to go through food of all the four seasons to get well.

I soon realized that I did not acquire asthma overnight. I had built it moment by moment, hour by hour, day by day, month by month and year by year. How? By not knowing the principle of eating hearty, tasty, nutritious meals of vital live foods—natural, pure and whole—in harmony with the body. Yes, I had my share of coffee and donuts and I also had my share of the result!

After three months, the physical part of me was pretty well taken care of, and I was prepared to return home and maintain a good nervous system, a good bloodstream, good circulation and get the proper exercise and rest. Also, my motivation had been stirred, and I found my attitude changing. My mind and heart were opening.

After I left Dr. Jensen's Ranch and returned to my home in Bremerton, Washington, I was still taking Prednisone about every two weeks. I felt like a "Prednisone junkie" because I couldn't get off of it. Now, I realize that I lived in fear that I had to take the drug in order to breathe, and that very fear kept me in chains.

I lost five pounds during each asthma attack. The lessons I had learned at the Ranch about mental attitude were slipping away. I lived and relived Dr. Jensen's lectures. Recalling the Doctor's advice that we need to read and learn about all things, I began to look into homeopathy. I was fascinated by it and when I learned of a young medical doctor who practiced homeopathy, I went to see him.

This doctor prepared what homeopathists call a constitutional remedy, and around April 1, I took my first dose. After eight days, I began to wheeze and cough up an abnormal quantity of phlegm. (I believe I manufacture more mucus than anyone in the world; too bad it can't be converted into gasoline!) Two days passed and the mucus stopped flowing.

The least exertion brought on labored breathing. Day and night hot water packs were applied to my back over the lung area, and this brought some relief. Onion packs were applied to my chest and back. A vaporizer was running around the clock.

Claustrophobia came up. I had a phobia of doors being closed, of small rooms, of being alone. I was afraid of becoming unable to breathe, tightness around my waist and even window shades being drawn at night.

I craved space, air and light but I had no energy and couldn't sleep. I began to feel like giving up. My bowel movements were the size of a pencil. Although the bathroom was twelve steps from my bed, I had to have assistance to get there.

Twelve steps seem as long as a mile when you don't have the energy to take them. Each step I had to wait for my breath to return. I had to be fanned.

Tedrol was given to me in place of Prednisone. The withdrawal from Prednisone was as bad as an asthma attack. I had adverse reactions to Tedrol and wanted off of it.

Sometimes the cure seems worse than the disease.

Because the main bathroom in my two-story house is upstairs, I went for days without even a sponge bath. I simply didn't have the energy to cope with the stairs. When I finally made it up there, I was faced with another phobia—water, of all things!

Looking in the mirror at my nude body, I was alarmed and appalled. I'm sure I ran a close second to the starving Cambodian refugees. The muscles of my upper arms and buttocks were flabby, weak, lacking in tone, sagging to the point where I could grab a handful of loose skin.

The scale showed my weight was 92 pounds. I looked like a skeleton, with my skin so drawn I could see every rib. Although I didn't know it at the time, many of my friends thought I was never going to make it.

I had to have help around the clock, because it was utterly impossible for me to function on my own. Asthma attacks seemed to occur around 4:30 pm and again at 1:30 am with coughing and raising of thick phlegm. Sometimes this phlegm was so thick, it stretched like bubble gum.

Many nights I tried resting with two or three pillows under my shoulders and head. I didn't know what it was like to have a good night and I rarely slept. Night after night, day after day, with tears streaming down my face, I repeated, "I feel wonderful...I feel wonderful." At the same time, I wondered if it would ever really come to pass.

My dear friend, Judy, assured me it would, so I kept on with courage. I remember Dr. Jensen telling me that during a crisis not even the doctor can do anything but offer moral support. That is the whole truth! The body knows its own strength and will pull you through when it is ready.

Before I started the homeopathy treatments, I enrolled in a psycho-cybernetics class and began to use thought projection which proved very beneficial. I told myself, "I know, I know, I know, that I can mentally see I can have all,depending on how far I want to go."

I read uplifting books and used the 24-hour telephone prayer line of our local Unity Church. Once in the wee hours of the morning when I needed help, I dialed the prayer line only to find it busy. Someone else needed it too. Praying for others in need and forgiving yourself are helpful in your own healing.

In Dr. Jensen's book *Nature Has A Remedy*, he advised using the same principle to bring a certain thought into mind to start each day.

"I am filled with health and the joy of living.
There is sunshine in my soul today.
The clouds have rolled away, and I feel
Confident, reassured—ever so confident.
I feel young, ever so young.
Every day in every way I feel younger and younger.
I feel like a new and wonderful personality,
And I can overcome everything
With the greatest of ease.
I feel Wonderful—Truly Wonderful!"

I am telling you here that it really works!

At this period of my life, I am deeply moved by what growth in consciousness has accomplished for me. I can truly say that asthma has been a real blessing and I know the needle isn't stuck in the problem any more. I have my eyes on the solution instead of the problem. My potential is unlimited. The answer to our problems lies inside us and is so difficult to find and learn.

As I gained strength I began to exercise as I was taught at Dr. Jensen's Ranch, but also including exercises on the easy jogger and the slant board. I purchased an exercise machine on which I pedal twelve miles each morning. I had a sandbox built so I could walk in it five minutes each morning. Soon I'll be walking in the grass. I exercise for five minutes on a narrow bench with two 6-ounce plastic bottles filled with sand to expand and develop my chest. Morning and night I skin brush for five minutes.

Since learning of Norman Cousin's use of laughter to heal his body, I laugh while exercising and get a big lift out of it! Laughing is said to massage the liver, exercise the chest and recharge the medulla of the brain.

I never let myself get fatigued. I've learned to drop everything and rest for 30 minutes to an hour. I listen to my body's needs.

When I was staying at the Ranch, my tongue was heavily coated. Every morning now I stick out my tongue just to see how beautiful it looks and to remind myself to think of and bless Dr. Jensen. He says he is in the healing process all the way with his patients and he really means it.

The bathroom scale now says 113 when I get on it. My muscles are firm, my skin has good tone and I no longer carry flabby tissue. I am no longer the droopy-winged chicken of Bremerton, Washington. For the first time in several summers, I will be able to wear short-sleeved and sleeveless garments.

Best of all, my friends are catching on to this new way of life. Several of them and I took a course in pendulum polarity, and we now teach it along with the program of nutrition exercise and food for the mind and spirit in accordance with Dr. Jensen's teaching.

I have learned so much from Dr. Jensen. I learned that the body is ready for change when we are ready. I learned that age makes no difference. I could start anytime I wanted to start. The body is a servant to the mind. Treat the body well and it responds, and what the body needs comes out of the garden through the kitchen.

I learned the skin was the largest organ of the body. I had thought the skin just covered me. I found out that I had to take care of it—that my skin had to breathe, too. The Doctor's teachings and philosophy appealed to me, and I realized I was going to now get an education instead of medication. Not only did I learn about the skin but learned that I had to get in and take care of the bowel activities. I had not realized that the bowel and the bronchials were so closely related. I never realized anything was wrong and no one had said anything about it.

"Al-Fal-Fa," I learned, means the Father of all Foods and is one of the best foods one can take for the bowel. I learned that a lazy bowel does not move bulk along very well. Alfalfa tablets are made up of the fiber or the bulk of the leaf of the alfalfa, and this gives the weakened bowel tissue something to exercise on. It gradually becomes stronger. The chlorophyll in the alfalfa tablets helps to develop the friendly colon bacteria, getting rid of odorous gases, and is a good food for the friendly bacteria. The tablets must be cracked before swallowing. Alfalfa has ten times the mineral content of most grains.

I had made everything so difficult when it was so simple. All I needed was the knowledge of all these wonderful things that our Creator put here for us. Our bloodstream is out there in the gardens...in the fruits, vegetables, nuts, seeds, sprouts, herbs, berries and chlorophyll.

Chemical shortages cause diseases. Greens should be the basis of our meals. They make up for many of the shortages in elements we have every day. The greens will help keep cooked vegetables and meat from putrefying and spoiling in the colon.

I had lived on substitutes for over 60 years. I went back to nature; but I had to earn each step. I really had to dig. But I had grown ready for it through desiring a new way of life so strongly that conditions and circumstances had to yield.

It is truly a wonderful feeling to breathe deeply and not hear a rattling of mucus. Every morning upon arising and every night before retiring, I do deep-breathing exercises for seven minutes. Deep breathing helps bring new materials for building the cells.

I have been able to observe through my iris photographs the healing crises working and developing. It is very impressive to see the white healing signs replacing all the dark ones in the iris fibers. I have been through many, many healing crises, and after each one, it feels like another step upward to renewed strength and good health. It's a good, good feeling. I will never return to the old habits of eating.

My life has been enriched and blessed with the teachings and services of Dr. Bernard Jensen. The way of return to good health is not easy, but I like the results...I like living again!

I wanted to tell this personal story with the thought that perhaps someone who is struggling with asthma and respiratory problems will see it and know there is an open door to walk through to a new way of life!

This is probably one of the most difficult of all the cases that I have encountered and what made it difficult was the settlement of suppressants and toxic materials. Also the vitality and energy levels had been exhausted for many years.

In cases like this, it takes from one to five years to rebuild the body, but we find here a very diligent patient and one who was willing to work and earn her way back by very faithfully following a good physical program, as well as mustering together all her spiritual background. She needed much hope and a peaceful way of life. Everyone who is sick must have a good mental attitude for any replacement therapy to be successful in the body. Physically, it has been a matter of constant elimination of toxic materials and waste, going through a transition from the old to the new, and almost literally putting "new timber in an old house"—refurnishing a new circulation system.

A Patient from Maryland

When I first came to see Dr. Jensen in 1975, I couldn't even walk across the room unless I had my inhaler handy. Then I could take a breath and continue walking, again having to take another whiff before I was even halfway to my destination.

Originally, I met Dr. Jensen through a friend who suggested that I read his book *You Can Master Disease*, so I would have some idea of what his program was all about. When I finally went to see him at his Hidden Valley Health Ranch, I was in the process of trying to get off the drugs, but I was having a very, very hard time with severe drug withdrawal.

I was off junk foods from the moment I arrived at Dr. Jensen's Ranch—no more packaged foods, no more canned foods, no more fried foods and no more quick meals.

Of course, I changed my diet completely. For example, I was taken off bread. At one time, I thought that if I had a slice of bread and butter with a cup of something hot to drink that this would help my asthma! After I ate and drank, I was able to cough up mucus, thinking the bread and hot drink were helping to release it. I never realized that the bread was creating mucus and building more problems for the future.

When I changed my diet, it wasn't just in little things. It was a complete and tremendous change. I started eating more raw foods until about 80 percent of my diet was raw. I started drinking juices, especially carrot juice. The only cooked foods I remember eating those first few weeks were baked potatoes and steamed beets.

The retracing process was not easy. Dr. Jensen told me all the toxins and residues in my body would have to come out before I could get well. I also remember his lectures on mental attitude. They brought out the fact that you cannot get well if you're angry or resentful. And this proved really helpful to me in trying to change my attitude. I had made up my mind that I was going to be the best patient Dr. Jensen ever had. I was sick of being sick. It was hard to change lifetime habits, but I stuck it out. I would say it took me a good year to feel even 50 percent better and then another year to feel 100 percent better.

Some years ago, I had an operation on my lungs. At that time, I was having a great deal of phlegm and catarrh coming up every morning and all during the day. The phlegm was filled with pus and

I was very short of breath. The doctors took all kinds of tests and X-rays. They poured oil down my nose and took a picture of the lungs. Then they put a tube down into the lungs and took pictures from the inside. The consensus of opinion was that I had bronchiectasis, a deep-seated infection of the left lung. Bronchiectasis is defined in the *New American Medical Dictionary* as "A dilation of the small bronchial tubes often associated within the lungs."

The doctors said that if I didn't get that lung section removed, it would just get worse and worse as I got older. They advised surgery. I consented because I didn't know any better at the time, but if I had known then what I know now, I would never have had the operation. That was 26 years ago. Instead of getting well, asthma set in right after the operation. It's true, I did not have the deep, thick pus that I had before the operation, but instead, I developed a condition that made me feel more dead than alive for 23 years.

My life was centered around going from one doctor to the next. One winter, I had five different cases of pneumonia besides the asthma—all in one year! So you see, the operation did not cure a thing and neither did any of the drugs I was taking. They didn't relieve anything because I still had asthma after taking them. Then I went on to have other drugs and other health problems.

One of the conditions I had was colitis. This condition existed for 10 years before I went to see Dr. Jensen. I was unable to have any raw foods, raw salads, raw fruits or vegetables. I missed them so much! Everything had to be cooked. I had indigestion a great deal of the time and constipation as well. But I paid hardly any attention to that because my asthma was so overwhelming that my full attention was on it to the exclusion of everything else.

When I arrived at Dr. Jensen's Ranch, he put me on a new diet and a new way of living. I told him, "I'm not going to be able to eat! It's going to make me sick because I have colitis!!" Dr. Jensen said, "Let's just take one day at a time and see how things go."

Well, to my utter amazement, the colitis completely left after the five weeks of my first visit to the Ranch. And with my digestion I never had another bit...not even a speck...of trouble. Without any problem at all, I could eat all the raw fruits and vegetables and drink all the raw juices I wanted.

Now the wonderful thing about all this is not just what the new diet and way of living did for me, but what it did for my husband as well. Before I left for the Ranch the first time, my husband told me that if I learned a better way to live and benefitted from it, he would follow the new way with me. My husband had a heart condition, a bladder condition, for which he had taken a lot of antibiotics, a great deal of arthritis, the start of a prostate condition and a couple of spells with high fevers. The arthritis especially troubled him and often he would take eight different pills a day for it.

When I went to the Ranch and learned various things through Dr. Jensen's lectures, I would write a letter to my husband about what I had learned. To my great surprise, he started putting all this into practice right away. One of the first things he did was stop drinking coffee. He stopped eating citrus fruits because Dr. Jensen had said citrus fruits were usually picked green. Then when I came home, he went on the exact same diet I had followed at the Ranch.

Now he no longer has a heart condition. At one time, he was taking three different drugs for this problem. He had fibrillation of the heart which was very, very frightening. His pulse became so wild and erratic we couldn't even count it, so he was rushed to the hospital where they gave him an I.V. and drugs to slow the pulse down. But not any more—no more heart drugs and no more heart condition! Also, he no longer has a prostate condition or arthritis.

When I returned home, I can't say that all my difficulties were ended. I was cautioned concerning how long it would take to completely recover from the condition I was in. The air pollution in Baltimore, I believe, caused a shortness of breath which made it a constant struggle to breathe. But even a trip to the mountains didn't bring much relief.

My strength began returning over a period of months, but I still had a slight fever every afternoon as well as assorted other symptoms.

In early December, my fever went up to 102 degrees and I couldn't urinate or move my bowels. I went to a urologist who removed almost a quart of urine from my bladder. He thought I should feel great relief. Mentally, of course, I did. Physically, I still felt a pressure. Numerous tests were taken, and all were negative— there was no infection, bladder showed good tone, normal capacity, etc. The doctor was puzzled at my report of continuing pressure, but there was nothing he could do. I went home December 8 (my birthday), reassured but with no change in symptoms.

At home, I developed a pain in the side of my neck, the left side worse than the right. It felt like the blood vessel running down my neck was engorged and painful. I rubbed it gently, It lasted two days.

The next day I had pain in my left ear where I'd had three infections many years before. For some reason, this was accompanied by pain in both my upper arms. This lasted a couple of days. That same day I began to eliminate a bloody wine-colored liquid. I ignored it, and it stopped in two-and-a-half days.

Dr. Jensen had told me what I might expect during a healing crisis, but it is one thing to talk about it and another thing to experience.

I continued to sleep only fitfully at nights, waking every 45 minutes to an hour to urinate. Since I knew my bladder was fine, I tried to ignore it. I had a malodorous discharge all this time, but crazy as it sounds, I wasn't sure where it was coming from. I had told the urologist about it, and of course, he should have checked it at that time, but he didn't. I was wearing sanitary pads. They had such an unbearable odor they had to be removed immediately from the bathroom when I changed them.

Weak, feverish, lacking appetite, I forced myself to eat, but my weight still dropped to 101 pounds. The pressure sensation on the bladder and constipation continued.

Finally, I saw my gynecologist. He immediately identified what was on my sanitary pad as pus and said I must have an abscess. After the examination, he said, "It definitely is an abscess, but you've done the job yourself. It's open and draining." The doctor said the abscess was the cause of the pressure sensation and prescribed Erythromycin as a precaution. I decided to take it in hope it would ease the pressure.

That was a terrible mistake. I took 1,000 mg of the drug for four or five doses and became sick. I became nauseated and felt as if I couldn't get enough air. I couldn't eat. I spoke to the doctor who reduced the medication, but I decided to cut it out entirely.

The awful discharge continued, the pressure continued and the sleeplessness continued. The constipation remained, and I marked time each day. When I returned to the gynecologist, he said the abscess would probably continue to drain another two weeks. "Isn't nature wonderful?" he asked, telling me to continue the antibiotic. I just nodded.

Three days later the discharge turned pink, and I realized some sort of turning point had been reached. I called the doctor who said it was okay.

My appetite improved, and my weight went up to 104 pounds.

As the abscess continued to drain, my gynecologist puzzled over what could have caused it. "If you had a diverticulum," he said, "it could have perforated and drained through the bowel wall into the pelvic area." Dr. Jensen had told me I had diverticula when he examined my irides!

Well, I look at it as having had the bowel pocket cleaned out. Once it healed, the doctor could see the two holes where the drainage had come from. I distinctly recalled my first visit to him, when he examined my sanitary pad, and it smelled so foul that he asked the nurse to take it out of the room.

It seems hard to believe, remembering back, how thick and profuse the discharge was. I could feel it running out of me like a faucet. Sometimes I would put on a fresh pad and it wouldn't be sufficient to absorb the flow, so my clothes would get soiled. Altogether, the abscess drained from November 25 to January 20. All that time, my stomach was blown up like a balloon even though my weight was low. When the discharge stopped, my stomach began to come down.

During those weeks, I spent a lot of time on the slant board to alleviate that terrible, ever-present pressure in my lower abdomen. Walking helped when I wasn't too weak. But most of the time I just lay on the couch or in bed with a heating pad on my abdomen or back. The heat helped. Later, I began taking colemas.

When I began taking colemas, the water only went up the colon a short way and mostly water came out. Now I can feel it all the way up and across to the right, and I am having very good results. I still can't make a bowel movement unless I skip the colema that day, but I'm sure that will work out. I don't worry about it.

I've also had pains which were diagnosed 30 years ago as neuralgia, but I ignore these, too.

In order to change we sometimes have to break completely away from our old ways of doing things...even from family customs and family menus. My children have said they admire their father and me very much for what we have accomplished. They don't know anyone else in our age group who has completely changed their way of life. My husband and I feel so well and so wonderful, we're just thankful for each and every day now!

I now weigh 120 pounds and don't really want to gain anymore weight. Everyone tells me I look 15 years younger. My walk is rapid and springy and I feel great. I sleep like a top and rarely get out of bed to go to the bathroom. My breathing is perfect! I never use a handkerchief. It's absolutely wonderful to breathe freely!

If I could give advice to others based upon what I've been through, the first thing I would tell them is what someone once told me, "If you have the good fortune to know of a person who can teach you a new way of life, then go to that person to learn." But if you are not able to go to see someone like Dr. Jensen, **then you must** cut out of your diet all foods that are not good for the health. You must eat live food, food fresh from the garden that is raw and you must always strive to eat the whole food. You must get plenty of rest, sunshine, exercise and good fresh air...and, of course, no sugar, no smoking, no drinking, no coffee and no tea except herb teas.

There is a lot to be said for eating live foods. If you take a carrot or a potato and keep them at home, the potato will grow from the eyes and the carrot will grow greens out of the top. These are live foods...they have life in them and can give life in return for rebuilding your body.

When I returned home after my first visit to the Ranch, my husband told everyone he had gotten back "the girl I married." This was a wonderful compliment for me to hear, because when I first came to Dr. Jensen, I was suffering just like a little old lady. Now I am just fine and take no drugs at all. Recently I was visiting friends and had a fever. My friends told me to take an aspirin, but I said, "No, indeed! I'll just get into bed, take some distilled water and by tomorrow, I'll be well." And that's just what happened; by the next day, I was well.

Very important too is one's mental attitude. You have to find a new way to approach life mentally as well as physically. People have told me that the reason I got well was because I believed in Dr. Jensen. But that is really not the entire truth, because I believed in the medical doctors too when I went to them. I believed that they wanted me to be well; however, I did not get well.

When I changed my way of living and ate what was whole and alive, then that also helped to change my mental attitude. I found out that what feeds my body also feed my nerves and brain cells so I could develop a different outlook on life. When you're sick, you're in a mental rut and it's very difficult to get out of it.

Now everything is different...I'm able to take care of the house and even the grandchildren! My daughter-in-law is sick and I'm able to take over and help out with the children so she can get well.

During those years of my own illness, I never would have believed it possible that I could again do such a thing! But I am doing it today.

The sad thing about giving advice is that most people are not ready to listen even though it's so simple. They just seem to enjoy their own way of living, as well as taking all the medicines that go with it. I guess they expect the doctor to cure them, but I have found out through experience that it cannot be done that way. You have to live a different life in order to get well. I positively believe that the job for the doctor of the future will be to teach people how to get well and stay well.

RESPIRATORY CONDITION CASES

Interview No. 1

Dr. Jensen: J.P. has been feeling very good. He originally became our patient about eight months ago. He's been living a very good life and all at once, he has hit a period...after feeling his best...that the lung structure seems to be throwing off considerable catarrh and mucus. He calls it "almost liquified smog." He has had a consistent cough for the past two or three weeks.

He has been bringing up really dark-brown material. He hasn't had too much trouble with that in the past, so it's hard for him to believe that this could come on after feeling so good. But this is where the typical crisis comes in. It usually comes after a person feels his best. The bowels are good right through this healing crisis.

You had a little bit more gas through the last week or so compared to before?

Patient: Yes.

Dr. Jensen: Alright. You have lost a couple pounds. You've been going through with chiropractic treatments, and even they are not too effective right now through the healing crisis, because the healing crisis is your own body making the changes. In fact, you can't do too much about it, and no doctor can predict or tell when— say the moment or the hour—that you're going to have this healing crisis. You really can't predict it. You have these crises when you're supposed to—when your body builds up enough energy, then throws it off. You do live outside Los Angeles, don't you?

Patient: Right in Los Angeles—North Hollywood, "Heart of Smog."

Dr. Jensen: Well, this is the bad aspect. I've often mentioned that it's hard to get anybody well in Los Angeles. It's hard to keep clean here from a lung standpoint. Looking into the iris of the eye, we find considerable darkness through the left lung structure. And we find there's quite a white elimination process going on in the bowel on the descending colon, but there is also a complete change in the left lung structure, and this is the reason we call it a healing crisis.

This is an elimination process—this is when the catarrh gets on the run. We're sorry for the pains, aches, troubles, but this is typical of an elimination process. You mentioned that you sounded almost like a tuberculosis patient. Well, the coughing has sort of let up now.

Patient: Yes. The coughing hasn't really bothered me the last week.

Dr. Jensen: I think now that you're over the hump. I think you have another week of recuperation. Energy is low. If you don't hit too many late hours...give yourself a bit of rest for another week or so...you'll find you will come out of this very well. We like to have a change in patients and you are a changed patient. All you want to know is where you're going and most patients do. So when this comes about...this is a time when you don't do anything. You try to take care of your good health—and try to do everything for the good of your health, having the right diet as much as possible. Just do the right thing now and you'll find in another week or so that your body will be built up and you'll be in better health than you've been in many years.

I think you're over the elimination period. You don't need to worry about elimination anymore. Go right onto your regular diet, and a regular diet as we have given it to you will be half elimination and half building. Your elimination is really over. You don't need to go too much more on it. I only say that when the elimination period comes, like you're in now, use broth and fluids for a few days.

You will find that this elimination will be a bit more complete as you liquify that catarrh and get it on the run. Go right on into your regular diet and add those extra juices—vegetable juices especially. Don't have too much of the fruit juices even though this is the fruit season. Stay with six vegetables and two fruits a day. And I'd like to hear from you in two weeks. In two weeks you should feel right on top of the mountain again.

Patient: Thank you. You're the most incredible doctor I've ever seen. I've lived on nose sprays. Bronchitis two or three times a winter. That's why I got into health foods, trying to beat that. But since I got into being a vegetarian, eliminating pasteurized dairy products and all that stuff, I can't remember my last cold. Must have been three or four years ago.

Dr. Jensen: You see, we're following what we call Hering's law of cure, and that is, we cure from within out, from the head down and in reverse order as we have built it up in the body. You're bringing back some of your old problems. And while you might have been having them over a period of years, in the healing crisis we concentrated on elimination. And it really hits you hard. You followed a typical path of what we call "suppression." I'm glad to hear about the problems you had in the past, because I had to bring them back in order for you to get well.

Patient: Okay. Thank you again.

Interview No. 2

Dr. Jensen: How old are you?

Patient: Turned 34 the first of July.

Dr. Jensen: Thirty-four...still a young lady. Let's have a look in your eyes. Well, we have lymph gland congestion here. This means an excess of catarrh, phlegm and mucus flowing from the bronchial tubes into the lymph glands. We have bronchial and lung catarrh. This is one thing we have accumulated over a period of years. This is mostly on the left side.

We have two pockets in the bowel on the left side that are causing a little disturbance. We have a couple of pockets over on the right side. Now these pockets are not bad at all—the ones on the left side are the most important. And we have a scurf rim, which shows the skin is not eliminating acids as fast as it should. The kidney on the left side is a little underactive.

We have lovely healing signs in the bowel area and in the bronchial tube area. There are beautiful healing signs even in the kidney area. The adrenal glands have some nice healing signs. And with the healing signs in the adrenal glands, the integrity of the tissue, that is, the rejuvenation ability is much better. That holds the vitamin C and gets rid of infection and that gets rid of catarrh, phlegm and mucus better than it did in the past. Possibly there's been more silicon added to the diet and the chemical balance is much better here. And you should be ready for a healing crisis, a good elimination process. Have you had many colds?

Patient: I've never had a great deal—I've had one or two a year. Since taking vitamin C over the last six years, sometimes I'll go a whole year or just have one in a year.

Dr. Jensen: But then you took the vitamin C to keep from getting the colds.

Patient: Well, I just put it in my diet as a regular thing...also for my nose.

Dr. Jensen: How's the energy?

Patient: Well, I've been having a really heavy time teaching this summer—a heavy schedule. I'm a little tired, but at the same time, I go out to play volleyball or do a few other things I wouldn't have six months ago. I'm tired, but active.

Dr. Jensen: Yes...how about lately? Have you had any elimination process of any kind?

Patient: I've been experiencing one since last week. Mostly a lot of stuff from the nose—heavy mucus and worse on the left, definitely.

Dr. Jensen: Worse on the left side?

Patient: I've already cleared up on the right, but the left is still hanging on. It's been over a week.

Dr. Jensen: That's interesting, because I find more trouble on the left than on the right. I was wondering if you had a sinus disturbance. This is just draining of the head area.

Patient: Well, yes, it's been heavy drainage. Really quite a lot.

Dr. Jensen: Quite a lot? Really blowing the nose? Coughing too—a bit in the morning?

Patient: A little bit, a lit bit of a cough, never too heavy, but still there. No soreness in the pleura area.

Dr. Jensen: No, but the cough was there for getting rid of the congested catarrh that wants out. Well, I feel it's all for a good purpose; it's a cleansing process. You've asked for a clean body, so that's what goes along with it.

Patient: I accept that; it's for the good.

Dr. Jensen: Alright. You were feeling pretty good before it happened though, weren't you?

Patient: Yes, I was feeling great.

Dr. Jensen: Well that's when it usually happens. It's just after they say they feel good.

Patient: I was feeling good, quite on top of it. Then I got hit with this.

Dr. Jensen: As far as I'm concerned, it's the best thing that could ever happen to you, because I work for these healing crises, and it's hard to believe that you should have one right in the middle of summer. Nobody has colds and things. Why should you have one?

Patient: Well, it had something to do with my program.

Dr. Jensen: Well, see, catarrh is a word that means "flow." Through liquidation, bringing this catarrh to a liquid state, it begins to flow. And it always comes after a person starts living better. You added more exercise to your program?

Patient: Yes.

Dr. Jensen: You've been trying to live a better life, cutting down on the junk foods?

Patient: They're pretty much off limits. Sometimes I'll have a little treat; but I'm sticking to the diet.

Dr. Jensen: Less sugar?

Patient: Yes, but only pure sugars. My friends are recognizing that if I go out with them we have to go someplace where I can order the right foods, or if I go someplace, I have apple juice with them. I want to have my own integrity about what I'm doing.

Dr. Jensen: Wonderful. The bowels are good?

Patient: Yes much better; very regular, daily. Sometimes it was a strain before, but now it isn't.

Dr. Jensen: You'll find that usually the bowels are good when we go through a healing crisis, a healing process, such as you're going through. You're like an old sponge, and we're squeezing out the toxic material and dipping it into some nice clean, clear water. You're going to come out clean and that's what you want.

Patient: Earlier you were speaking about the scurf rim. Should I be brushing my skin more often than once a day?

Dr. Jensen: Once a day is enough, especially in the summer, you're outside more and wearing less clothing. Now that it's summertime we can cut down on some of this. In fact what I'd like you to do is just take the alfalfa tablets, digestant and rice bran syrup. Silicon for the nerves. Silicon helps to keep catarrh on the go. Be sure and have the four morning supplements: rice polishings, flaxseed meal, wheat germ and sesame or sunflower seed meal. When it's cooler weather, take a little vitamins A and C, to keep up and to compensate for some of these past problems and the inherent weaknesses.

Patient: Fine. Keep up with the slant board. Right?

Dr. Jensen: Yes, my dear, this is part of your daily program.

Patient: It has improved my circulation, I know that.

Dr. Jensen: Alright. We'll see you in another five months.

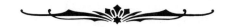

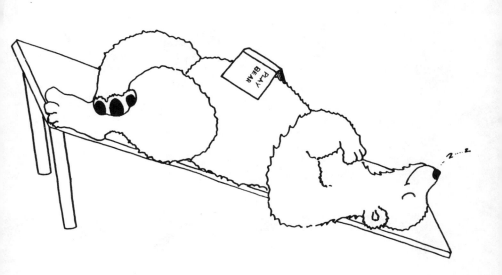

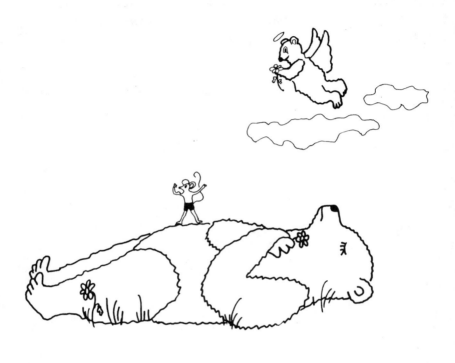

"Happy Hunting in a New Country!"